Lose
Those
Last
10
Pounds

Also by Denise Austin

JumpStart

Hit the Spot!

Denise Austin's Ultimate Pregnancy Book

Lose Those Last 10 Pounds

The 28-Day
Foolproof Plan
to a Healthy Body

Denise Austin

BROADWAY BOOKS   New York

To my Mom, Jeff, Kelly and Katie,
who set the "tone" of my life every day with their love

BROADWAY

LOSE THOSE LAST 10 POUNDS. Copyright © 2000 by Denise Austin. All rights reserved. Printed in the United States of America. No part of this book may be reproduced or transmitted in any form or by any means, electronic or mechanical, including photocopying, recording, or by any information storage and retrieval system, without written permission from the publisher. For information, address Broadway Books, a division of Random House, Inc., 1540 Broadway, New York, NY 10036.

Broadway Books titles may be purchased for business or promotional use or for special sales. For information, please write to: Special Markets Department, Random House, Inc., 1540 Broadway, New York, NY 10036.

BROADWAY BOOKS and its logo, a letter B bisected on the diagonal, are trademarks of Broadway Books, a division of Random House, Inc.

Visit our Web site at www.broadwaybooks.com

Library of Congress Cataloging-in-Publication Data
Austin, Denise.
    Lose those last 10 pounds : the 28-day foolproof plan to a healthy body / Denise Austin.—1st ed.
        p.   cm.
    ISBN 0-7679-0469-9
    1. Weight loss. 2. Reducing diets—Recipes. I. Title: Lose those last ten pounds. II. Title.
RM222.2 .A92 2000
613.7—dc21   99-049879

FIRST EDITION

Fidget-cize photographs by Doug Sanford
All other photographs by Kelly Campbell

00 01 02 03 10 9 8 7 6 5 4 3 2 1

Contents

Acknowledgments

I am always so grateful to my mom, who brought up all five of us kids with endless energy and dedication. And to my dad for teaching me that discipline and perseverance will make things happen.

To all my sisters and my brother, who are my biggest fans. It's so great to have such a close-knit family!

To my husband, Jeff, who is so supportive of me. You always give 110 percent . . . you're the very best. Thank you for everything. To my two daughters, Kelly and Katie, whom I love every second of the day. I cherish being a mother more than anything in the world—it's a constant joy!

I want to thank Stacy Whitman and Wynne Whitman for their crucial contributions to this book. Together (as sisters always are), they really "shaped" this book. You were a joy to work with. Thank you!

I am so happy to thank Bob Asahina, my editor . . . it's great to have you back! And many thanks to Ann Campbell for your editorial expertise. A big thanks to Jan Miller, my literary agent, who is so smart and so fun.

A big thanks to Leslie Bonci, R.D., for your help with planning such nutritious meals . . . and thanks to Rita Calvert for "cooking up" some great recipes.

Special thanks to Daphne Howard and Darren Bell for all of their help.

I also want to thank all the people who come up to me, no matter where I am, and tell me such wonderful things about how I helped motivate them and helped them feel better. Thank you! Knowing that I'm truly helping other people is what keeps me going.

Lastly, thank you to all my friends, both professional and social, for helping me along the way.

Introduction

CONGRATULATIONS and welcome to a new world of better health and fitness—without those extra 10 pounds you've been carrying!

By picking up this book you have just taken the first important step to a new lifestyle filled with countless rewards: a healthier body, more energy and a great new shape. And since you have made the first move by purchasing this book, I want you to know that from here on in, I'll be with you every step of the way.

Whether you need to lose 10 pounds or 50 pounds, the program here is a great beginning. We're going to work together to develop new health habits for the present and for the future—and help you slim down to the shape that you desire. *I* know you can do it; now *you* need to believe in yourself. Remember: You can have all the money, material possessions and friends in the world, but without a healthy body, it's tough to enjoy them. Consider the next 28 days an investment in yourself—one that will lead to a lifetime of better health and happiness.

If you're wondering why I'm writing this book, it's because people like you have asked me to do it. Each week I receive over *400* letters from all over the country, more than half of which ask for my advice on how to lose those last 10 pounds. Your written questions and feedback help me understand your feelings and concerns, so I can deliver the best possible information and advice to help you reach your goals. Now I'm sure there are a few skeptics out there who are thinking that I've never had to drop a pound in my life, so how can I possibly relate to you? Not true. As you'll read later on, after each pregnancy I had as many as 25 pounds to lose—and the last 10 were always the hardest. So I *can* relate to your situation. Even now, I work hard every day to stay in shape and to keep those pounds off. The good news is, I've found the secret to weight-loss success, and I want to share it with you.

In this book I'm going to teach you everything I know about losing weight, getting fit and changing your life for the better. After 20 years as a health and fitness professional, I have seen every fad, diet and crazy scheme for losing weight. But I've also seen what works, and I've streamlined these techniques in the program presented here. I'll help you to lose body fat in a healthy way—so you don't regain it over the long term. Together we're going to "rev up" your metabolism by eating right and exercising. I'm going to help you burn calories whether you're working out, sitting in a car or cooking dinner. No longer will you have any excuses to skip exercise. By incorporating exercise and movement into your daily routine, you can boost your energy, reshape your body and take off those unwanted pounds—and KEEP THEM OFF!

Best of all, with my plan, if you lose, you gain better health! Losing just a few pounds can dramatically affect your long-term health picture by lowering your blood pressure and cholesterol levels. By maintaining a healthy weight, you can reduce your risk of heart disease, certain cancers and diabetes. Losing weight may even help you reverse some of the damage caused by carrying extra pounds. Best of all, you'll feel better! You'll look younger, have more energy and gain confidence. The quality of our lives is amazingly affected by healthy eating, exercise and a positive attitude. Once you get a handle on these three things, everything else falls into place—including your personal relationships, your job and how you feel about *you*. You'll discover that a healthy diet can be delicious and satisfying. As you burn fat and build muscle, your body will actually decrease in size and shape. In four weeks, you'll notice that your favorite clothes not only fit, but that you look great wearing them.

This book provides you with a basic weekly framework and all the tools you need to get started. It includes 28 days' worth of meal plans and recipes. I've even added some extra recipes for you to mix and match—and to help you after the 28-day program is over. We'll work week-by-week and focus on the big picture, so you won't have to weigh yourself every day. I'll share with you my secret ways to sneak exercise into your day as well as my favorite cardio, stretching and toning exercises. I'll also explain what works for me and how I manage to stay fit with a full-time career, a husband and two young daughters.

As you'll soon see, you don't have to starve yourself or become a marathon runner to lose weight. By making a few simple but effective lifestyle changes, you can watch those 10 pounds melt right off. My fat-busting plan can work for you—whether you are a man or a woman, fit athlete or former couch potato, have just turned 20 or are celebrating your silver anniversary, have always carried a little extra around the middle or just had a baby and are eager to get your old shape back. It's for anyone who wants to get energized, feel good about themselves and get more out of life.

Now that we know what you stand to gain—and lose!—by embarking on this program, don't wait another day. Let's get going!

Part 1

Getting Started

1 | Personalize Your Program

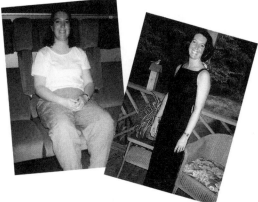

Sarah *dropped 35 pounds in time for her 10-year high school reunion. Her family and friends complimented her on how wonderful she looked. "Denise, you have helped me to look and feel better about myself—thanks for your motivation."*

There is only one you. You are unique in every way, from your fingerprints to your sense of humor, and from your reason to lose those last 10 pounds to how you need to do it. I created this plan as a framework for all of us. But since we're all different, you and I need to work together to develop your own individual weight-loss plan. The first thing that we need to do is figure out where you are and where you need to go. Read the scenarios presented here and take some time to find the one that most closely applies to you. This way, you'll be able to focus on your specific needs as we work together over the next 28 days.

Situation 1: You have a big event coming up . . . a wedding, a reunion or vacation to a sunny place.

Your goal is set: You need to fit into a snug bridesmaid dress. You hope to look "exactly the same" at your high school reunion. You want to throw on a bikini instead of shorts and an oversized T-shirt when you hit the beach. And you have just four weeks to make it happen!

First, let's get your priorities straight. For the next four weeks, you need to stay focused on your goal. This may mean making substantial changes to your routine. I'm going to ask you to devote at least half an hour a day to exercise. You'll have to say a loud "No!" to temptations like rich desserts and alcohol. You may have to spend less time watching TV and more time planning healthy meals. Or you may have to make other concessions, such as going to bed earlier so you can get up in the morning to do your workout. But trust me—the end result will be worth it!

A month before I begin the filming schedule for my television show, I really start watching my diet and exercising more. I know that in a few short weeks, I'll be putting on a leotard and stepping in front of a camera. And we all know that the TV camera can make a few extra pounds look like 10. So donuts are out and longer workouts are in. Although it might be difficult at first, I'm always happy later—and usually I'm happy during, too. When I eat well and exercise regularly, I'm full of energy and confidence. And you will be, too.

To stay focused on your goal, keep imagining yourself without those extra pounds you've been wearing—and with a tighter tummy and more muscle tone in all the places you want it most. Post positive reminders (phrases like "You can do it!" or "You deserve to feel good!") on your refrigerator, your calendar and your desk at work. Remember that every minute you exercise brings you that much closer to your goal. Let your loved ones and coworkers in on your plan and ask for their help. A good support system is often the key to successful weight loss.

No matter how anxious you are to shed those last 10 pounds, don't do anything drastic like starving yourself. Extremely low-calorie fad diets may help you drop some weight fast, but the weight you lose will be water and muscle tissue. By the time your big event arrives, you probably won't have the energy to enjoy it. You won't have done a thing to firm up those flabby areas. And you're almost guaranteed to gain back the weight as soon as you start eating normally again.

Your goal may be to fit into a new dress size for a particular event, but I want you to fit into that new dress size forever. If you follow the steps presented in this book, you'll learn new habits to help you lose and *keep* the weight off. You'll feel (*and* look) so good at the end of four weeks that you won't want to go back to your unhealthy habits. I promise!

Situation 2: You've already lost some weight but have hit a plateau.

Talk about frustrating! You've lost 15, 20 or maybe even 30 pounds and dropped a dress or a belt size or two. Then all your progress seems to trickle to a stop, and the scale gets stuck about 10 pounds above where you want to be.

Weight-loss plateaus happen for different reasons. In your case, you've probably been following the same routine for too long. You've been consuming the same foods day in and day out, and your exercise program hasn't changed since you started working out. The good news is that your body has adapted to it and learned how to do it more efficiently. The bad news is that since your muscles aren't working as hard as they did in the beginning, you're burning fewer calories with each workout.

Don't quit now! Getting past a plateau can be tough—but it can be done. You just need to shake things up and give your metabolism a little kick. You can begin by making changes to your diet. While my eating plan encourages you to experiment with different foods, you can also try changing *how* you eat. Smaller, more frequent meals are key, as they enable you to keep your body constantly fueled throughout the day—without overdoing it. Whatever you do, DON'T SKIP MEALS! Depriving yourself of calories causes your metabolism to slow down and will ultimately defeat your efforts to reach your target weight. We'll discuss this more in chapter two.

To keep your body burning as many calories as possible, you need to keep your muscles guessing. The program in this book is designed so that you never do the same aerobic workout twice in one week. If you decide not to follow the aerobic workouts I've provided, try creating your own mix-and-match schedule. Do my *Sizzler* video one day. Another day, ride an exercise bike, go swimming or play tennis. On the next day, jump rope, climb stairs or take a power walk. Make it your goal to stimulate as many different muscle fibers as possible.

If you have a favorite workout that you love, you don't have to abandon it. Just mix things up a bit by changing your intensity, time or tempo. If walking is your thing, try changing your routine a bit. Walk hills. Add a few minutes of slow jogging. Really pump your arms to get your upper body involved. Take a long, slow walk one day and a short, superfast walk the next. Throw in some skips or jump up and touch a tree branch (when no one's looking, of course).

In Chapter 2, I'll discuss interval training—a fabulous fat-burning workout. If you've been exercising regularly and are in relatively good shape, this could be the ticket to jump-starting your metabolism. If you're just launching an exercise program, you'll need to build a solid fitness base before getting into interval training—it's intense, and doing too much too soon can create unhealthy stress on your bones, joints and muscles.

You've worked hard to get where you are. Now the key is to work *smart*. You may resist change at first, but give it a try. You'll be surprised at how fun and liberating it can be. You're close to your goal . . . just hang in there!

Situation 3: You have 20 or more pounds to lose.

You're probably thinking that this book is just for those lucky people who have to lose only 10 pounds or less. Not so. Whether you need to lose seven pounds or 47 pounds, you have to start somewhere—and this book is the perfect place. Why? My plan is designed to create healthy eating and exercise habits that will last a lifetime. No matter how much you have to lose, you need to do it safely and effectively. It's the only way to do it without experiencing a rebound.

Since you have more than 10 pounds to lose, you're going to have to work longer than 28 days—but believe me, you'll be happy you did. I know it's difficult and intimidating, so pace yourself by focusing on small goals. Use my plan to lose 10 pounds, then do it again, and again, and again, until you've reached your ideal weight. Small goals are wonderful, because they allow you to measure your success. With every 10 pounds you lose, you'll feel better and better. And if you feel great, you'll want to keep going! You'll change your habits to include more fruits and vegetables in your diet and less fast food. As you become stronger and more fit, change your routine regularly by adding intensity and interval training to help you avoid a weight-loss plateau. You will have a newfound awareness and respect for you body and your health, and I promise you, the weight will come off.

Recently, my mom needed to lose 20 pounds. The weight had crept on over the years—and because she had high cholesterol, high blood pressure and a family history of heart disease (her father died of a heart attack at age 44), she knew that she had to trim down. At first, she felt overwhelmed and kept putting it off, so I encouraged her to begin by setting her goal at 10 pounds—and she did. By cutting back on junk food and exercising more (she did my Lifetime TV show *Denise Austin's Fit and Lite* every weekday morning), she was able to lose those first 10. Even better, her cholesterol went down 20 points. So did her blood pressure, and she was able to cut her blood pressure medication dosage in half. She felt so encouraged that she's decided to keep going and try to lose the remaining 10.

The more weight you lose, the more fun you will have incorporating movement and exercise into your daily routine. Don't get discouraged when you first start exercising. If you walk half a mile every day for a week, the next week you'll be able to walk three quarters of a mile, and eventually a whole mile. Exercise

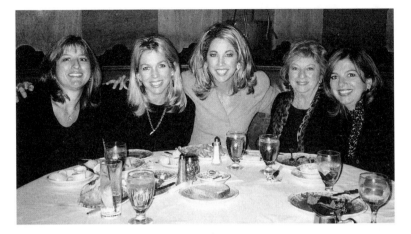

Here I am with my sisters and my mom: Donna (eight months pregnant), Anne, me, my cute little mom and Kristine. We love being together, especially eating!

will become increasingly easier, and before you know it you'll be following along with the exercise plans I've outlined. Remember: Losing the first 10 pounds deserves as much applause as losing the last 10!

Situation 4: You're a new mom.

First off, let me say congratulations! Motherhood is a truly joyous experience. From the moment you feel the first kick inside of you, you learn the meaning of unconditional love and understand what life is about. But it also can be a bit of a shock. Suddenly it feels as if you have a new body, and you wonder whether you'll ever get your old one back.

You *can*. I know—I've done it twice. With each of my pregnancies, I gained 35 pounds. By the time I left the hospital, I'd lost only 10 pounds and my belly was so big and mushy that I looked as if I had another baby on the way. I had 25 pounds to lose and a lot of work to do to get my tummy back to its usual size and shape. The pounds slowly came off—and the last 10 were the hardest. But with a little sweat and perseverance, I was successful.

Whether you had your baby two months or two years ago, you can be successful, too. Personally, I think it's best to start losing the baby fat soon after delivery. Otherwise, it's easy to let the extra pounds accumulate. But you still can lose the weight and reshape your body, even if your "baby" is now a preschooler or even a teenager. It's *never* too late to get started.

The four-week eating plan in this book provides good, balanced nutrition for both nursing and non-nursing moms. If you *are* breast-feeding, you'll need to add 500 extra calories a day; when your baby's relying on you for sustenance, you don't want to cut back on calories too much—and breast-feeding burns 300 to 500 extra calories a day. To support your milk supply, aim to get those extra calories from calcium-rich foods such as yogurt or cheese (see list, pages 257 to 258).

If you're a brand-new mom, you should get your obstetrician's approval before beginning an exercise program. With vaginal deliveries, most doctors recommend waiting two to four weeks to resume full activity. If you had a C-section, you should wait a little longer—maybe starting with slow walks at week four and slowly building up to full activity after six weeks. Always listen to your body; don't do too much too soon.

Of course, your abdominal muscles will be in serious need of attention. Tightening your tummy after having a baby is no different from doing it any other time—you just need to start slowly and be patient! In this book, you'll find some of the best postpartum abdominal exercises, such as the Reverse Crunch (page 163) and the Basic Crunch (page 163). As with everything else, consistency is key. Once your doctor gives you two thumbs up, begin doing crunches every day, then gradually work in other abdominal exercises.

If you have a newborn, your next question will probably be "But *when* will I find the time to exercise?" My answer: You have to grab every chance that you get—and there are more chances than you realize. When I had my two precious girls, Katie and

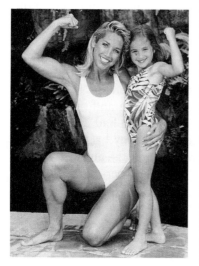

Kelly, I would do toning exercises during their morning naps. Twice a day, I would put them in a carriage and go for half-hour walks. Once your baby is about four months old, you can also put him or her in a baby jogger and do one of my 30 exercise videos or my morning show on Lifetime.

It won't always be easy. But keep reminding yourself that you're doing something good for both you and your family. Exercise will give you energy so you'll be better able to handle the demands of being a new mom. You'll teach your baby and any

Here I am "flexing" with my daughter Katie; she's another me. . . .

other children the importance of good health habits. Plus, you'll feel better about yourself—and you'll pass those positive feelings along to your kids!

Situation 5: You've gained 10 pounds because you quit smoking or are recovering from an injury or surgery.

If you just quit smoking, you get my hearty congratulations! You have just taken the single biggest step toward improving your health. Smoking causes more than 400,000 deaths in the United States each year; you would have to gain 100 to 150 pounds after quitting to make your health risk equal to what it was when you smoked. So don't let the extra pounds you've gained tempt you to light up again. My fat-busting plan can help you return to your former weight while controlling your cravings for nicotine. The key? Exercise. Instead of reaching for the lighter, walk around the block, go for a jog or walk up and down the steps at your office. Your body will release endorphins that elevate your mood and make you feel better—the same thing a cigarette used to do. Since nicotine is an artificial stimulant that helps keep you going, exercise—a stimulant—is an excellent substitute.

Many former smokers gain weight because they replace cigarettes with food. One of my metabolism-boosting strategies is to eat more often, so you satisfy your need to go from hand to mouth with healthy snacks like celery sticks filled with peanut butter, juicy apple slices, watermelon chunks or bowls of crunchy cereal. Be sure to stock up on good-for-you snacks both at home and the office, so you don't end up reaching for fattening junk food if a nicotine craving strikes. You can refer to the daily meal plans listed later in this book for more ideas.

Are you recovering from an injury or surgery? Then chances are you've simply been sedentary for too long. Your body has forgotten how great it feels to move and exercise. Once you get your doctor's OK, you need to start slowly and do what you can at your own pace. If you've suffered an ankle injury, for example, concentrate on upper-body exercises while you build up strength in your ankle. If you can't do one particular move, pick another—don't use your injury as an excuse to skip exercising. Check with your doctor or physical therapist to find the exercises that are suitable for you and do them regularly. The most important thing is to keep moving in whatever way you can. You may not be able to do it all, but don't let that stop you. You can still do it—I know you can!

As we move forward, keep your special needs in mind. I'll remind you of what's best for your specific circumstances, but only you know your real limitations. My plan is designed to meet the needs of many people. You can pick and choose what feels good and what works for you. Instead of being restricted to a dull diet and boring routines, I want you to explore all the different food and exercise options and see how great they make you feel. This will be your pathway to better health . . . and a better body.

Next stop—revving up your metabolism!

2

Your Formula for Success

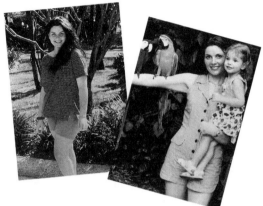

Lisa *wanted to lose the 10 pounds she had gained during her pregnancy and did it by using my 28-day program.*

By this time, you're probably wondering when we are going to get to this basic framework I keep referring to. Well, here it is! Once you understand what the program entails, I'll explain why it's so important to incorporate it into your weight-loss agenda. Here's what's going to happen:

- You'll keep your metabolism supercharged by eating three balanced meals and two snacks—including lots of fiber-rich fruits and veggies.
- On Mondays, Wednesdays and Fridays, you'll do 30-minute aerobic workouts. You can choose your favorite activity or follow my planned workouts for each day.
- On Tuesdays and Thursdays, we'll spend 30 minutes toning and firming up with a variety of weight training, yoga and Pilates Method exercises. (The Pilates Method, created by Joseph Pilates, who trained dancers in the 1950s, involves lengthening and strengthening floor exercises that focus on the abs and torso.)
- Saturdays are Play Days—my favorite! You'll do at least 60 minutes of swimming, biking, tennis, even gardening—you name it.
- Sundays are Free Days. Take the day off, or, better yet, use this day to do something fun—try a new sport, take a stroll

through a new part of town or treat yourself to an hour of yoga and meditation.

• You'll burn hundreds of extra calories each day with "Fidget-cize"™. This term may sound strange, but you'll see what I mean later in this chapter. "Turn idle time into toning time."

• You'll increase your flexibility and combat stress with my five-minute Mind-Body-Spirit routine on Mondays, Wednesdays and Fridays (or whenever the spirit moves you).

Why This Program Works

You may look at the photo on the cover of this book and think to yourself, "She's so lucky . . . she doesn't have to worry about her weight. She must have been born that way." I only wish that were the case! Rest assured that I have to work at keeping my figure, just like everyone else. But I will admit that staying fit became much easier once I learned how to keep my metabolism revved up 24 hours a day. This is the simple secret to successful weight loss.

What exactly is your metabolism? It's the rate at which your body burns calories for fuel. The higher your metabolism, the more calories you burn. It's that simple. There are several factors that determine your metabolic rate, including your eating habits, how physically active you are and how much muscle you have.

Now, it's true that certain people are born with faster metabolisms than others. That's why some folks seem to eat whatever they want and never gain an ounce, while others barely look at food and seem to pile on the pounds. Your metabolism also tends to slow down as you age, mainly because you lose muscle and become more sedentary.

Fortunately, you *can* change your metabolic destiny for the better by making a few simple lifestyle changes. You also can change it for the worse by crash dieting.

There are two *natural* ways to boost your metabolism: eating and exercise.

When you severely restrict calories or skip meals, your metabolism slows down to conserve fuel—your body's way of protecting itself from starvation. Any weight you do lose is from deterioration of muscle tissue and water loss, *not fat*. As soon as you return to your regular diet, you will gain, *gain, gain* back the weight you lost—and often more.

The latest fad—the high-protein diet—isn't much better. With protein diets, you restrict your intake of energy-boosting carbohydrates and eat more protein and fat. While you may lose weight, it's because you're consuming fewer calories—not because of some magic nutritional formula. Since most of the weight that you lose is water, you may find yourself dehydrated, tired and dizzy. When you up your fat intake, you may increase your risk of heart disease. And you can only guess what occurs when you reenter the real world of bread and other starches— which is destined to happen since they're nearly impossible to avoid. The calories add up quickly and the pounds pile back on— especially if you're not exercising.

There are two basic components to a successful weight-loss plan: healthy eating and exercise. The key word here is *and*. You need to move to drop those last 10 pounds. Why? Countless studies show that cutting calories alone does not result in long-term, permanent weight loss; my own nonscientific study shows the same thing. If you're not burning calories through exercise, you'll have a hard time creating the calorie deficit necessary to lose weight—and as I've mentioned before, you need muscle to maintain a vigorous metabolism. I've seen it work for my friends, my family, my viewers and me. It will work for you as well!

Ready to give your metabolism a makeover? Let's do it!

The Importance of Exercise

DENISEOLOGY
The indisputable key to long-term fat loss is exercise.
*It's a proven way to boost your metabolism
and increase caloric burn.*

OK, I'll admit it: Exercise can be a drag. But don't imagine for one minute that I'm suggesting that you don't have to do it—you do! For every reason you can think of *not* to exercise, there are a million better reasons why you should—more self-esteem and lower risk of cardiovascular disease (the number-one killer of both men and women), to name two! There are plenty of mornings I'd rather sit on the couch and eat donuts with my kids. But I know how much better I'll feel after exercise and all the wonderful things it will do for my body and my state of mind. Even if I struggle through the first five minutes of my workout, my body almost always starts to loosen up and I get a second wind. By the end, I feel like a new person!

WHAT'S STOPPING YOU?
How to Overcome Exercise Barriers

Work deadlines, parent-teacher conferences, diapers, errands—it's easy to let our busy lives get in the way of regular exercise. First step: Identify your exercise obstacles. Then find ways to deal with them one by one. Here are some simple solutions to get you started:

Problem: I don't have time to exercise.
Solution: Who does? We need to make exercise a TOP PRIORITY! Successful exercisers make workouts integral parts of their daily routines. So schedule daily appointments with yourself (write them down in your day planner or on your calendar!) and treat them as you would a doctor's appointment or business meeting—you're going to be there, no ifs, ands, or buts.

Problem: I have to take care of my family.
Solution: Plan fitness activities that include your kids—ride a bike, play kickball, go ice-skating, bowl or throw an impromptu dance contest in your living room. If you have a little one, use a baby carrier and climb stairs or power walk at your local mall.

Problem: I'd rather spend time with friends.
Solution: Make exercise a social activity. Organize a mixed-doubles tennis match, recruit friends for a hike or long walk or join a local bicycle club with your buddies.

Problem: I'm too tired.
Solution: OK—then just exercise for five minutes. You owe yourself that. Chances are, though, if you make it through five minutes, you'll make it through 10, and before you know it, your whole workout! Those first five minutes are always the hardest, but you'll be amazed at what you can accomplish once you start. You can avoid lethargy by making sure you have plenty of fuel—grab an energy-boosting snack like graham crackers, low-fat yogurt or a banana.

Problem: I'm just not motivated enough.
Solution: Find an exercise buddy. Research shows that having a dedicated partner makes you more likely to stick with an exercise program. You won't skip your power walk or date at the gym if your friend is waiting for you on the corner! Afterward, you'll feel doubly great because you not only had a great workout, but you also overcame procrastination. It takes a little effort, but you can do it!

Step 1: Burn the Fat!

Anyone who wants to lose 10 pounds and live a long, healthy life *must* participate in some form of cardiovascular exercise (anything that gets your heart rate up for at least 15 minutes). Cardio activity is vital to burning fat and keeping your metabolism in high gear. A 30-minute kickboxing workout, for example, can burn up to 400 calories. Even better: Your metabolism stays charged for up to *two hours* after your workout ends, so you continue to burn more calories without lifting a finger!

> Get moving and start doing, and your mind will follow.

Fat burning aside, you need aerobic exercise to keep your whole system running smoothly. A fit and well-functioning heart is at the center of a healthy body, and exercise makes it strong. A strong heart then benefits your entire body by pumping fresh oxygen and nutrients to every last organ, cell and muscle.

As you saw earlier, all I'm asking for is three 30-minute aerobic workouts during the week. This is what I personally do, so I know it works. You can do the fat-busting workouts I've provided on pages 167 to 176 or pick your own. Having flexibility in your exercise routine keeps you moving, motivated and burning that fat. So for a change of pace, try any of the metabolism-boosting activities listed below. My only request is that no matter what the activity, you keep it up for at least 30 minutes.

SUPERCHARGED CARDIO WORKOUTS

Power walking	Aerobicizing (either a class
Jogging	or a video)
Running	Rowing
Cycling	Kickboxing
Swimming	Jumping rope
In-line skating	Using an elliptical machine
Cross-country skiing	Dancing
Stair climbing	

Exercise doesn't have to be a chore! And to prove it, you're going to plan a fun activity for the weekend that will keep you moving for 60 minutes—walking barefoot on a beach, playing tennis, cross-country skiing, ice-skating, playing basketball or biking with your kids. Or, if you need to multitask, try mowing the lawn, gardening or even cleaning your house. Remember that exercise = movement.

You don't need a pair of gym shorts or exercise shoes to have an effective workout!

This program encourages you to try a host of different exercise methods. Variety is crucial to keeping both your muscles and your mind stimulated. When you do the same exercise routine day in and day out, your body starts to adapt by essentially "memorizing" your workout. The aggravating result: Your muscles don't have to work as hard, so your progress levels off. Eventually you start burning fewer calories with each workout.

Over the years, I've received thousands of letters from people saying that they exercise three days a week but haven't lost weight. When I ask them what they do for exercise, most of them say, "Walk." Walking is an excellent workout, but if you walk the same route at the same speed day after day, your body will start to plateau in as little as eight to 12 weeks. Anyone who wants to drop some weight or have firmer thighs, arms or tummies will have to make a few changes and get beyond their established routine to see results.

Which leads me to interval training—one of the best fat-busting workouts around. With interval training, you alternate high- and low-intensity spurts of exercise. For example, you'd do three minutes of walking followed by three minutes of jogging, and then continue to alternate your pace throughout your entire workout. Many types of exercise adapt to intervals; try doing interval sets on a stationary bike, a stair climber or a rowing machine. Because you really get your heart rate up, an interval workout burns more calories than an even-paced, moderate-intensity workout—and your metabolism can stay elevated for up to *four hours* after you stop! More on this topic in the opener to my walk/jog interval workout on pages 145 to 146.

A cautionary note: Interval training isn't for everyone. At least not right away. If you've never exercised before, or it's been a

THE POWER OF 10

There are lots of days that I run out of time and just can't fit in a full workout. What do I do? I do what I can—even if it's just for 10 minutes. It is hard to believe that 10 minutes will do any good, but it does! According to research conducted at the Cooper Institute for Aerobics Research, you get almost the same health benefits if you split your daily 30-minute quota into three 10-minute bouts per day. Another study from the University of Pittsburgh shows that people who exercise in 10-minute spurts may exercise more overall than those who strive for 30 minutes. While your goal should always be half an hour of straight cardio, a 10-minute workout is definitely worth the effort in a pinch!

while since you have, you'll need to build up gradually. For the next four weeks, you should stick to low- to moderate-intensity activities, such as walking, jogging or easy cycling. Don't do too much, too soon. You'll only end up discouraged and sore. It's more important to exercise consistently than to push yourself to exhaustion once a week!

Remember, if you hate it, you're not going to do it. So find an activity—or activities—that best suits your lifestyle and your schedule. Keep experimenting with different workouts until you find one you love—or at least one you can live with. While variety helps keep your calorie-burning potential at a max, it's always better to do *something* than nothing. What you do is never as important as just doing.

Step 2: Build the Muscle!

Everyone is looking for that elusive, magic weight-loss trick, whether it comes in the form of a pill, a new fad diet, or an expensive sheet of plastic wrap that you sleep in. People always ask me if these things work. My response: Don't kid yourself! The only "magic" weight-loss trick I know of is strength training—weight-bearing exercise designed to build and strengthen your muscles.

> A regular and consistent workout program preserves and builds muscle mass. Even at rest, muscle burns almost twice as many calories as fat. ▼

Muscles work miracles on your metabolism. For every pound of muscle you add, you automatically burn an extra 35 to 50 calories per day. The reason? Muscle demands more energy than fat does. Therefore, the more muscle you build, the more calories your body burns. In one study from the University of Rhode Island, women who lifted weights twice a week saw their body fat drop more than 2½ percent, while their nonlifting counterparts didn't lose any.

In this program, we're going to work on building muscle two days a week. One workout will consist of traditional weight-training moves—push-ups, squats and bent-over rows. You'll need a pair of dumbbells for that one. The other will feature softer, yoga- and Pilates-inspired exercises that are designed to build strong, flexible muscles. These moves use your own body weight for resistance, so no equipment is required.

Keep in mind that conditioning your muscles doesn't mean bulking up so that you look like Arnold Schwarzenegger. It does mean burning more calories and giving your body a whole new shape. Your arms and legs will look and feel firmer. Your waist will become narrower and your belly will shrink. Your clothes will fit better. You'll start to look younger and feel stronger!

Even if you've never exercised before or aren't used to working with weights, you can do my twice-a-week toning workouts. They don't require a gym membership or fancy machines. In fact, if you don't have the basic tools listed below, you can use items that you probably already have around the house:

> 3-, 5- and 8-pound dumbbells (for the 3-pound weights, you can substitute full soup cans or water bottles)
> 1- or 2-pound ankle weights (optional)
> A weight bench (substitute a sturdy chair)
> A jump rope
> An exercise mat (optional)

Don't forget: Building muscle is a must-do when it comes to losing weight. So even if my toning exercises aren't your favorite part of the program, you need to do them if you want to lose those 10 pounds and look your best. You'll love the results—both how you feel in your clothes and how you look in the mirror!

Step 3: Get Flexible!

Stretching is a wonderful way to start your day—it's how I greet every morning. The second I get out of bed, before reaching for a glass of juice or turning on the TV, I do my five-minute Mind-Body-Spirit Routine to wake up, get in the right mind frame and get rid of those early-morning kinks. It's one of the greatest gifts that I give myself.

The stretches in my Mind-Body-Spirit Routine aren't like the ones you did in your eighth-grade gym class. They're based on holistic traditions such as yoga, Tai Chi and QiGong. They're designed to help build long, flexible muscles, increase your circulation and provide the peace of mind that's essential for a healthy, balanced life.

This is probably the part of this program that you'll be most tempted to skip. You're not burning lots of calories, so why bother, right? Wrong. Building flexibility is crucial as you age. When you stretch, you pump blood carrying

Stretching helps you become more aware of how you feel, both inside and out. Stretch away the ouches and the stress!

vital nutrients to your muscles and tendons, which keeps them healthy. New research conducted by strength expert Wayne Westcott shows that stretching also helps to build muscle—and as we know, that translates to a faster metabolism. And then there's the spiritual aspect. As you flow from one move to the next—drawing your consciousness inward through deep breathing—you'll be able to tap into your inner reservoir of positive energy as you let go of the negative.

You can do my Mind-Body-Spirit Routine first thing in the morning, before or after your workout, or in the evening to rid yourself of pent-up stress from the workday. When I'm on the road, I like to do it right after a tough photo shoot or publicity event—before heading out to a business dinner. At home, I sometimes do it after putting the kids to sleep—it helps me make the transition from "go, go, go" to "time to go to bed." Best of all, you can do this routine *anywhere*.

Try to add it into your mix at least three times a week. The whole routine takes only five minutes, and you'll notice a difference almost immediately. As the blood and oxygen pump through your body, you'll feel more energized and alive. Your legs, back, neck and shoulders will loosen up, relieving aches and stiffness. You'll lengthen your muscles, which will give you a longer, leaner look, especially in your thighs. You'll feel calm and connected rather than tense and rushed. If you're feeling anxious or uptight about something in your life, this soothing routine is a fantastic remedy.

At the end of each daily workout, I've also provided a few soothing cool-down stretches. When you stretch, you release toxins from your muscles that have built up during your workout and send nutrient-rich blood to your joints. A post-workout stretch will also help keep your muscles supple, so you don't feel sore and you minimize your chances of injury. Talk about a wise time investment!

Step 4: Fidget-cize!

Like most of you, I love to eat. But if I'm going to eat the way I like to, I know that I've got to keep moving constantly and burning those calories off. I'm not an exercise fanatic—with a full-time career and two kids, I can't be. In fact, as I mentioned earlier, I do only 30 minutes of "official" exercise a day. My secret: making every minute count and sprinkling mini-workouts (I call it "Fidget-cize") throughout my day.

Don't laugh. Fidgeting works—and there's research to prove it! In a study conducted at the Mayo Clinic in Rochester, Minnesota, a group of volunteers, ages 20 to 35, was fed 1,000 extra calories a day for eight weeks. At the end of the study, some participants had gained as much as 16 pounds while others gained as little as two. The difference, researchers say, was fidgeting. The people who gained less weight tended to be restless—constantly standing up and stretching, shifting around in their chairs or tapping their toes.

> Little quickie exercises can have a bigger impact than you realize on your weight, your energy levels—and even ▼ your brainpower!

Even small movements burn calories that might otherwise be stored as fat!

There are other benefits, of course: By getting up and moving, you improve your circulation, especially through your lower body and legs, where blood tends to stagnate. Increasing your blood flow can give you an instant energy boost! It can also help combat sluggishness and make you more mentally alert, whether you're trapped behind a desk or in an airplane seat.

I never miss an opportunity to move, even when I'm watching TV or am stuck in rush-hour traffic. During commercial breaks I do easy toning exercises, like triceps dips and ab crunches. If I'm stuck in a traffic jam, I hold on to the steering wheel and do tummy tucks. When I talk on the phone, I pace back and forth while I talk. When I brush my teeth or blow-dry my hair, I do squats or standing leg lifts. You get the idea—you don't need a lot of free time to burn calories.

I'm not a natural fidgeter, so I had to train myself to move. And that's exactly what you're going to do for the next four weeks. On pages 203 to 212, I've included plenty of ideas to get you started. If you can, do one Fidget-cize every hour on the hour. Sure, your coworkers might give you strange looks as you do Saddlebag Slimmers at the copy machine. Who cares? You're doing something good for you!

If you stick with it, Fidget-cize will soon be second nature. Suddenly you'll be burning hundreds of extra calories without even realizing it! All you have to do is walk, pace, tap your toes, squeeze your bottom, stretch your back or pull in your tummy. Even something as simple as getting up out of your chair will make you a better calorie burner. Let's start right now: Stand up and stretch both arms over your head; then march in place for five seconds and reach up and stretch toward the sky again. That's it! Pretty easy way to burn an extra 500 calories a day, wouldn't you say?

Eating Right

Remember all those crazy diets you've tried in the past? Only brown rice, only juice, only protein, only bean sprouts. Sure, you lost a few pounds, but where are those pounds now? They're back. As I mentioned before, crash diets set you up for failure because they trick your body into actually *conserving* fat. They are self-defeating, so *don't* buy into them.

The meal plan presented here *isn't* a diet. It's a new way of eating that will help you stay slim and healthy for the rest of your life. Not only will you learn what to eat, but you'll learn when and how to eat—equally important. Don't plan on following it for four weeks, then returning to your old bad habits. After you taste the gourmet recipes and see the great results, you'll want to eat this way forever!

This plan is terrific because it's simple, realistic and not ridiculously strict. With the help of top nutritionist Leslie Bonci, I've put together 28 days' worth of quick, easy recipes. At the start of each week, we've provided grocery lists so you can zip in and out of the store. And the meal plans include treats (yes, even candy bars and cookies!) so you won't have to deny your sweet tooth. Acknowledging these cravings is the only way you'll stick with the plan—and avoid gaining back the weight.

Fiber is the foundation of my fat-busting meal plan. Fruits, vegetables, whole grains and beans help reduce your risk of heart disease and certain kinds of cancer. Furthermore, fiber makes you feel full, so it's fabulous for whittling your waistline. Research conducted by the U.S. Department of Agriculture's Human Nutrition Center in Beltsville, Maryland, shows that fiber speeds food through your digestive system, essentially preventing your body from absorbing some calories. For each gram of fiber consumed, you can subtract about nine calories from your total calorie intake. By doubling your fiber intake from 13 grams (the average for most Americans) to 26 grams (the daily total in this meal plan), you end up deducting about 90 calories. You can boost your fiber intake even more by replacing lower-fiber snacks with the higher-fiber ones listed on pages 259 to 260.

On each day of this plan, you'll be consuming approximately 1,500 calories, divided as follows:

Breakfast—300 calories
Mid-morning snack—100 calories
Lunch—400 calories
Mid-afternoon snack—200 calories
Dinner—500 calories

As you can see, each daily menu includes three meals and two snacks. "Grazing" is an excellent way to keep your metabolism operating in top form. When you eat smaller, more frequent meals, your body processes food more efficiently, so it's less likely to get stored as fat. You also avoid sharp peaks and dips in blood sugar that lead to mood swings and binges. In addition, if your energy level stays up, you'll be less tempted to miss a workout.

This plan is about good nutrition, not deprivation or starvation! Your body burns calories more efficiently with a balanced diet, so each meal contains a healthy mix of protein (about 25 percent of total calories), carbohydrates (about 50 percent of calories) and fat (about 25 percent of calories). Men and breast-feeding women should plan to consume about 500 extra calories per day; simply boost your portion sizes slightly or eat a few extra snacks from the list provided on page 256.

For the rest of us, moderation is the key. So pay attention to the size of your meal. Servings in America get larger every day. No longer is a "large" big enough—fast-food restaurants and movie theaters are promoting super-size everything, from popcorn to ice cream sundaes. A fundamental part of this meal plan is a return to sensible portions. Use the following chart as a guide:

1 serving of meat, poultry or fish = the size of a deck of cards or a computer mouse (about 3 ounces)

1 serving of vegetables = a mound as large as a softball (about 1½ cups)

1 serving of starches and grains (cereal, potatoes, rice) = no bigger than a tennis ball (about 1 cup)

1 serving of fat (butter, olive oil, mayonnaise) = the size of your thumb (about 1 tablespoon)

1 serving of bread = a slice the size of a CD case

Another easy way to enforce portion control is to go for foods that come in single-serving packages. Little containers of raisins, baked tortilla chips, cereal and yogurt are easy to tote with you to work, school or even the beach. They may cost a little more, but they're one of the best ways to keep your caloric intake in check.

Now I know that over the next four weeks you're going to be eating at restaurants and grabbing food on the go. But just because you're not preparing your own meals doesn't mean that you're going to blow it! Simply watch your portion sizes and choose healthy, low-fat foods like the ones in the meal plan. Go for grilled meats and vegetables, avoid heavy sauces and order salad dressings on the side. Try to include a balance of carbohy-

HUNGRY? TRY THESE NATURAL APPETITE SUPPRESSANTS

- **GO FOR A WALK.** Research proves that a premeal stroll can help curb your hunger. Even better, it will give your metabolism a boost. So lace up those walking shoes and get moving!
- **EAT GRAPEFRUIT.** Citrus fruits contain an ingredient called pectin that helps minimize your appetite. (Remember the grapefruit diet?) So try squelching those late-morning or predinner hunger pangs with a grapefruit, an orange or a tangerine.
- **DRINK UP.** Water helps fill you up, so drink a big glass or two about 10 minutes before you plan to eat.
- **BRUSH YOUR TEETH.** If you're craving a postmeal treat, minty toothpaste will satisfy your sweet tooth, and your mouth will feel so clean that you won't want to nibble!

drates, lean protein and fat with each meal. If you're served a jumbo-size portion, ask your waiter to put half in a doggie bag right off the bat.

Since no one is perfect and no two days are the same, stay focused on the big calorie picture. There are days when you're going to slip. Maybe you'll fall prey to a slice of cake at a coworker's birthday party or you've just got to have a piece of your mother's gooey cheese lasagna. If this happens, don't get discouraged and give up. Just compensate by exercising a little longer or eating a little less the next day. As long as you even things out by the end of the week, you're still in great shape! We need to be flexible in everything we do—including the way we eat!

And yes, I'm talking about consuming alcohol, too. While alcoholic beverages haven't been factored into our fat-busting meal plan, you can treat yourself to a glass of wine once or twice a week. One 3½-ounce glass of red wine contains about 140 calories—and a 10-minute walk is all it takes to burn it off. But again, you want to practice moderation: Research suggests that alcohol reduces the rate at which our bodies burn fat. Also, when we drink, we tend to crave high-fat foods, such as chips and peanuts. So take it easy.

When you eat a balanced diet—as you'll be doing for the next four weeks—you can cover most of your nutritional needs. But it's always a good idea to take a daily multivitamin as an insurance policy. (I like Rexall Sundown.) Since most multiples don't contain 100 percent of the Recommended Daily Requirement for calcium, magnesium or folic acid, many experts recommend taking even more of those nutrients.

Maybe by now you're thinking, "Great! Four weeks of unin-

SMART EATING TIPS

It takes about 15 to 20 minutes after you begin eating before your body can tell that it's had enough. If you're a fast eater, you probably gobble down hundreds of extra calories before your brain gets the "No more!" signal coming from your stomach. Here are a few tips to help you slow down and savor each morsel:

- Put your fork down between bites and chew slowly.
- Eat meals with friends, family or coworkers and take the time to "catch up" between nibbles.
- Studies show that people are more likely to pace themselves if they play slow, relaxing music during a meal. So put on some classical music (my favorite is Bach) and nourish your mind while you're nourishing your body.
- Make eating purposeful, not an afterthought. It should be something you look forward to, not something you wolf down over the kitchen sink or on the run. Don't get distracted by the TV, phone or E-mail. Eating out of a bag, a box or a Styrofoam cup is sensory deprivation. Instead, take it out of the bag or container, put it on a plate or in a bowl, then sit down and soak in the colors, the smells and the tastes with each dainty bite.

---

spired, flavorless low-fat food." If so, you're way off the mark. As you'll discover in the next 28 days, healthy eating can be exciting, enticing and enriching—if you know what you're doing. Here are four basic tips for making each meal a satisfying feast for the senses:

1. Add Color. Variety is the spice of life, and it's also key to good nutrition! So consider the color wheel when you fill your grocery cart with produce. Then use splashes of color to decorate your plate. Instead of white rice, chicken and cauliflower, try chunks of roasted sweet potatoes, a swordfish steak and a spinach salad with cherry tomatoes. Throw snap peas, yellow peppers and bean sprouts into a stir-fry. Top yogurt with blueberries, banana and kiwi. Think Picasso!

2. Do Yourself a Flavor. Fat helps bring out the flavor in food. So when you're cooking low-fat, you'll need to replace the fat with lots of spices and other powerful flavors. Now's the time to become acquainted with your spice rack. Top toast or a baked apple with cinnamon, nutmeg, allspice or vanilla. Tantalize your taste buds with Thai and Indian spices, such as curry and cumin. Use fresh herbs, such as rosemary and basil, to jazz up pasta sauces. You can even start an herb garden on your windowsill!

3. **Munch and Crunch.** When you want to make a bland dish come to life, think of the four Cs—chewy, crunchy, crispy and creamy. To truly enjoy food, you need to experience every aspect of a meal, including the way it feels in your mouth. So toss a few nuts into a mixed green salad. Sprinkle Grape-Nuts onto a bowl of yogurt. Pair crisp celery and carrots with a smooth hummus dip. Texture adds a new dimension to food, so be creative!

4. **Aromatherapy.** Ever notice how the mere scent of freshly baked bread makes your mouth water? A meal that smells divine is always more satisfying. Here are some heavenly scents that will make you think "treat" instead of "tasteless," "blah" or "boring":

Fresh rosemary and other herbs
Garlic in olive oil
Freshly cut grapefruit
Raspberry tea
Lemon zest
A sprig of fresh mint

THE TOP 10 SUPER FOODS

Many Americans like to think that they can meet all their nutritional needs by popping a supplement. They shouldn't underestimate the power of Mother Nature! Real food provides us with countless benefits that you just can't get from a pill. Here is a roundup of 10 nutritional all-stars—plus some innovative ideas for working them into your menus.

Super food: Soy
Special power: Studies suggest soy can help reduce the risk of breast cancer, osteoporosis and heart disease as well as minimize "hot flashes."
Sneak-it-in strategies: Toss tofu into a stir-fry; crumble soy protein into pasta sauce; snack on yummy roasted or boiled soybeans; lighten your coffee with soymilk.

Super food: Tuna
Special power: The omega-3 fatty acids in tuna, salmon and other "fatty" fishes have been shown to help lower LDL—or "bad"—cholesterol levels and minimize menstrual cramps.
Sneak-it-in strategies: Toss canned tuna into a bowl of pasta; add it to a salad; put cubed tuna steaks and veggies onto skewers and grill.

Super food: Skim milk
Special power: Low-fat dairy products (think skim milk, low-fat

yogurt and low-fat cheese) are rich in calcium, important for building strong bones, teeth and muscles; they also contain potassium, which helps control blood pressure.
Sneak-it-in strategies: Drink a "skim" café latte instead of black coffee; add to a smoothie instead of juice.

Super food: Carrots
Special power: Bugs Bunny is no dummy: The beta carotene in carrots is excellent for your eyes, helps keep your arteries clear, and may prevent tumors from growing.
Sneak-it-in strategies: Snack on carrot sticks; add to canned soups; shred and add to sandwiches.

Super food: Blueberries
Special power: Deep red, purple or blue foods (think blueberries, cherries, strawberries, red cabbage, beets, raspberries, cranberries and purple grapes) contain phytonutrients called anthocyanins, which have been linked to lower heart disease and cancer risk.
Sneak-it-in strategies: Add to a smoothie; sprinkle over cereal or waffles; toss into a salad topped with raspberry vinaigrette.

Super food: Avocados
Special power: Yes, they're high in fat, but it's the "good," mono-unsaturated kind (meaning it won't clog your arteries). In fact, new research shows that avocados may *protect* against heart disease by lowering your LDL levels. Monounsaturated fats also help make your skin softer and your hair shinier.
Sneak-it-in strategies: Add slices to a veggie sandwich; stir cubes into chicken and rice soup; dip baked tortilla chips into fresh guacamole.

Super food: Spinach
Special power: Spinach and other dark, leafy greens are rich in bone-fortifying calcium; folic acid, which may help protect against heart disease and birth defects; and vitamin K, a nutrient necessary for proper blood clotting.
Sneak-it-in strategies: Stack onto sandwiches instead of lettuce; stir into hot soups; sauté with onion and use to top a baked potato.

Super food: Kiwi
Special power: One kiwi contains more vitamin C than an orange; it's also a good source of potassium, which helps keep your muscles functioning properly.
Sneak-it-in strategies: Cut in half and eat with a spoon; add slices to a bowl of cereal; use to spruce up a citrus salad.

Super food: Garlic
Special power: Eating half a clove daily can help guard against cancer; some studies suggest it also may lower cholesterol levels.
Sneak-it-in strategies: Sauté chopped garlic and green beans in olive oil; rub toasted bread with a garlic clove, then top with chopped tomatoes, onion and garlic to make bruschetta; poke holes in a chicken breast and fill with bits of garlic to flavor meat while cooking.

Super food: Broccoli
Special power: This cruciferous is packed with cancer-fighting nutrients such as beta-carotene, vitamin C, nitrogen compounds and sulforaphane.
Sneak-it-in strategies: Sprinkle finely chopped florets on pasta, rice, soup, salads or eggs; steam lightly and place in a whole-wheat pita with hummus.

Super food: Flaxseed
Special power: Flaxseed contains lignans and phytoestrogens that may help decrease your risk of cancer. Preliminary research suggests it also may help protect against heart disease.
Sneak-it-in strategies: Grind in a food processor or coffee mill and sprinkle on cereal, salads and yogurt.

3

10 Do's for Losing the Last 10

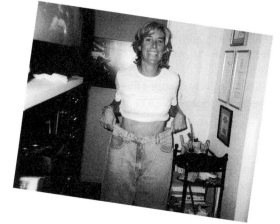

Beth lost the last 10 pounds in 28 days—along with four inches in her waist!

Don't eat this. Don't eat that. It seems like almost every popular weight-loss plan out there is filled with that dreaded four-letter word: DON'T. Not my plan! The most important word in mine is DO. The only way to lose those last 10 pounds and keep them off is to take a proactive approach to weight loss and add the following DO's to your daily routine. Even though you're anxious to get started, take 10 minutes to review these vital tips. The secret to your success may be found on the next few pages.

1. DO Keep a Food and Exercise Diary

Research confirms that writing down what you eat is one of the best ways to prevent poor food choices and useless calories. Two packets of sugar in your coffee, a spoonful of peanut butter, a handful of M&Ms from your coworker's candy dish—it all adds up. Perfect example: One of my friends is a chewing gum addict. She loves the stuff. But when she wrote down the number of calories per stick and the number of times she popped a piece of gum in her mouth, she was stunned to see how the calories added up.

Now I've already explained that my eating plan isn't meant to be ridiculously strict. I don't want you to deprive yourself of little pleasures or say, "Fattening foods are completely off-limits." But I *do* want you to be aware of where extra calories are coming from, and keeping track of what you eat is a great way to accomplish this. You'll probably be amazed at how many calories you're consuming—and identifying the real culprit foods is the first step in eliminating them. Once your metabolism gets going, those little nibbles, like gum, may not matter as much. For the next four weeks, however, you'll want to be careful.

Logging your workouts also can be helpful. When you look back and see your progress, you'll feel a sense of accomplishment and be encouraged to keep going. So take a few minutes to write down the details of each workout—how many miles you walked, how many tummy tucks you did, how long you stretched. Don't forget the little things, like walking down the street to mail a letter or climbing four flights of stairs. They count!

2. DO Get More Sleep

We hear about it everywhere—Americans don't get enough sleep. Unfortunately this can have serious consequences. When you're sleep deprived, you're more likely to catch a cold or have a car accident. Your work performance can suffer, too. But more important to our immediate cause, some research shows that a tired body is less efficient at building muscle and burning fat. You may go through the moves, but your sluggish pace makes your workout less effective. If you indulge in stimulants like cola or chocolate at this point, you add calories and sleeplessness to your unhappy body!

Sleep experts say that eight hours is the optimum amount of rest for most people, and my experience supports that belief. You should always aim to get *at least* eight hours a night—but especially during the next four weeks. To get my full eight, I go to bed early, around 10 P.M. If you have trouble adjusting to an earlier bedtime, turn the lights low and put on soft music one hour beforehand. Avoiding sunlight late in the day prevents excess stimulation. And drinking a little warm milk can help soothe you to sleep! If you have to give up *The Late Show* to get to bed at a decent hour, remind yourself that it's for a good cause—you!

3. DO Eat Breakfast

Although it may seem counterintuitive to weight loss, skipping meals at any time of day is a big mistake. You *really* need food energy in the morning to get your body moving. And I don't mean just coffee and a donut. Make breakfast well-rounded with a bit of protein and fruit as well as fiber. The simple act of eating wakes up your metabolism, so you start burning more calories right away.

What if you're not hungry when you wake up? Have something small—half a bagel, a glass of juice, a banana—just don't skip the meal altogether. You can train yourself to become a breakfast eater by starting off with small, snack-size meals. It takes us about seven to 10 days to adapt to a new habit, so by Week 3, you should be used to it, and even looking forward to your morning energizers.

Equally important is to get out of the habit of saving up your calories for an end-of-the-day feast. This not only robs your mind and muscles of needed energy throughout the day, it tampers with metabolism, which works much more efficiently if it has a constant, steady supply of fuel. As soon as you start withholding the calories your body needs to survive, it goes into the starvation mode we talked about earlier—storing as many calories as possible to ensure survival and thus keeping extra pounds firmly in place.

4. DO Strive for Five!

To lose weight—and stay healthy—you need to eat at least five servings of fruits and vegetables a day. They're low in calories, they give you energy, and they can help lower your risk of heart disease and cancer. Eaten raw, most fruits and vegetables are loaded with fiber, which, as we discussed in Chapter 2, helps you lose weight by blocking the absorption of fat and calories. Another plus!

Although many of us are not as friendly with fruits and vegetables as we should be, getting five servings a day is easier than you think. Portion sizes for fruits and veggies are much smaller than those of other foods, or the quantity of food generally scooped onto a plate. To get a full serving of fruit, you just need to eat half a banana, a small apple or a 6-ounce glass of orange juice. One serving of broccoli (approximately ½ cup) is the equivalent of two large spears. I easily eat three times that at any one meal!

You can find lots of innovative ways to sneak more fruits and vegetables into your diet. Some of my favorite strategies include: piling fresh spinach leaves, grated carrots or sweet red pepper onto a sandwich; tossing chopped vegetables into an omelet; adding frozen veggies to a can of soup; or throwing mango, banana or berries (or all three!) into my morning smoothie. For the next 28 days it'll be easy, since my meal plan is full of fruits and vegetables. In fact, I've **highlighted** them to show you just how painless it is to get those five servings.

5. DO Drink More Water

Water is truly the wonder drink. Everything about it is good for you. Water helps regulate your body temperature and keeps your digestive system performing efficiently. Your body needs water to flush out toxins—poisonous by-products from the digestive process. Water also breaks down fat, and your muscles need it to function properly and build strength. It also helps curb your appetite and makes your skin soft and supple.

Although eight to 10 glasses a day is the conventional wisdom, don't stop there—drink as much as you can. Ideally, you should consume 0.67 ounces of water per pound of body weight; for a 130-pound woman, that's almost 11 eight-ounce glasses a day. When you exercise, you need even more to control your body temperature and keep your muscles functioning—and you're losing fluid when you perspire.

Eleven glasses of water may sound overwhelming, but trust me, it can be done. How? Take water with you everywhere you go! Every morning, I fill up 5 water bottles for the day. One bottle stays with me at all times. The others get stored in my car, my office and my exercise bag. It takes a few minutes, but it ensures that water will always be within reach and helps me keep track of how much I drink. Once you get used to drinking water regularly, you'll find that you can't do without it.

If plain water is too boring for you and you crave flavor, try some of the low-calorie sport drinks or brew a quart of decaffeinated ice tea for a change. I also enjoy a glass of seltzer water with some fresh lime, lemon or a splash of grapefruit juice.

6. DO Eat When You Aren't Hungry

We all know that feeling of being ravenously hungry. Maybe you had to rush off to a doctor's appointment and missed lunch. Or maybe you got stuck in traffic on your way home from work and ate dinner much later as a result. As we've discussed before, skipping a meal, whether by accident or on purpose, is the easiest way to derail your weight-loss agenda. When you finally get your hands on food, you tend to overeat and fill up on quick-fix foods that are fattening and low in nutrients, like donuts, potato chips and ice cream. Afterward, you're stuffed and uncomfortable. You gravitate toward the couch. And exercise? Forget it.

I know it goes against everything you've ever been told. But to keep your body burning calories efficiently—and to avoid the binges that happen when you skip meals—you want to feed your body small amounts of food all day long. You won't ever feel starving—but that's a good thing. It means you're keeping your blood sugar levels on a healthy, even keel.

On a satiety scale of 1 to 10 (1 being starving and 10 being Thanksgiving dinner–type stuffed), always aim for a 5. Never let yourself get too hungry or too full. This may require some careful planning. Pack a bag of healthy nibbles to bring with you to work, such as carrot sticks, fresh fruit, cheese or soy nuts. Keep a supply of instant soups, graham crackers or cans of fruit at the office. Stock up on instant or portable breakfasts, like low-fat cereal bars or containers of yogurt, for days when you have to rush out the door. Always carry an energy bar or a package of Fig Newtons in your purse for fueling emergencies.

7. DO Get Moving Before Dinner

I like to go for a power walk or get outside and play with my daughters in the late afternoon or right before dinner. After a long work day, a quick walk along the Potomac or a rousing game of catch helps perk me up and releases stress. And that's not all: Research from the Cooper Institute for Aerobics Research shows that predinner physical activity—even if it's just a 10-minute walk—can help curb your appetite, so you end up eating less. Even better, it will give your metabolism a quick boost so your body is fully prepared for the food you're about to eat. So before you start preparing dinner, if you've already done your more extensive workout for the day, go for a short walk, hop on a bike, dance around your living room, do 10 minutes of yoga or try my Mind-Body-Spirit Routine (pages 213 to 217)—anything to burn a few calories and get your blood pumping!

8. DO Establish a Kitchen Curfew

Experts have different theories on whether eating in the evening makes you more likely to gain weight. I personally believe that it does, and here's why. During the day, you're constantly getting up and moving—lifting boxes at the office, running to catch the bus—so your body needs steady fuel. But by evening, your body starts to slow down as you return home and prepare for bed. Your metabolism slows down, too. Therefore, if you eat a large meal before going to sleep, the food is more likely to get stored rather than burned for instant energy. So when the clock strikes eight, turn off the lights and tell yourself that the kitchen is closed until morning. This will prevent late-night snacking and ensure that you won't be putting on pounds while you sleep.

9. DO Breathe

Your body needs oxygen to survive and thrive. If you don't get enough of it, your muscles won't function efficiently, and you'll feel sluggish and exhausted—a real hindrance to exercise and weight loss. So start each morning with three deep breaths—not your normal, everyday breaths, but deep, long, fill-your-lungs-with-air breaths. Then, throughout the day, every two hours, remember to take two more deep breaths. If you can, go outside, so you're breathing fresh, clean air. Open a window and stick your head out if you have to! Expand your lungs. Breathing is life . . . take your fill!

10. DO Smile, Laugh and Enjoy the Day

A lighter, livelier lifestyle without those last 10 pounds isn't just about doing push-ups and nibbling celery. To get lasting results, you need to focus on every aspect of your life. So while you work on changing your body, give yourself an attitude makeover, too. Remind yourself to smile more—make it the first thing you do

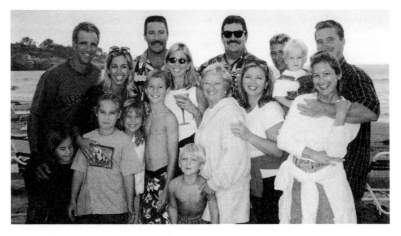

Me and my entire family at the beach enjoying our annual summer vacation.

every day. Let yourself relax and enjoy life's simple pleasures—a beautiful sunset, a bouquet of lilacs, a good book, a chat with an old friend. Take pride in your daily accomplishments and celebrate the healthy changes you're achieving. Make it a point to enjoy one big belly laugh every single day. Patch Adams isn't the only one who thinks laughter is good medicine: Many experts believe that it can boost your immune system and chase away the blues, and it will do wonders for your abdominals! Most important, try to actively appreciate all in your life that you have to be thankful for. You'll be surprised at how much lovelier the world is, and how much easier it is to achieve your weight-loss goals, when you bring a positive attitude to everything that you do.

Part 2

Your Fabulous Four-Week Plan

4
Week One

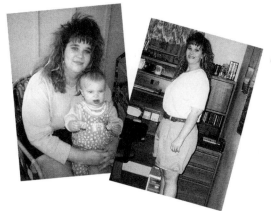

Kimberly lost 52 pounds in three and a half months on the program. "I am on my way to my goal—to lose 75 pounds! I couldn't have done it without you, Denise."

WEEK AT A GLANCE

MONDAY: Cardio—Walk/jog intervals (30 minutes)
Mind-Body-Spirit Routine (5 minutes)

TUESDAY: Toning—Weight training (30 minutes)

WEDNESDAY: Cardio—Fat-Burning Blast with light weights
(30 minutes)
Mind-Body-Spirit Routine (5 minutes)

THURSDAY: Toning—Yoga and Pilates Method (30 minutes)

FRIDAY: Cardio—Triple cardio mix with muscle-toning circuit
(30 minutes)
Mind-Body-Spirit Routine (5 minutes)

SATURDAY: Play Day (60 minutes)

SUNDAY: Rejuvenation Day

Now that you're familiar with your goals and our formula for success, let's get started! You're embarking on a challenging 28 days, but I know you can do it—today, tomorrow and the rest of your life!

Bear in mind that there's a lot of new information to absorb this week. You're going to be learning new ways of eating and exercising, so be sure to factor in a little extra time to do your grocery shopping, prepare your meals and learn your new workouts. You may even want to spend some time in the evening studying the next day's plan and preparing certain meals and snacks in advance. That way you can wake up in the morning with a clear agenda and jump right into your weight-loss program.

In terms of exercise, the format for each week is the same. As I've already mentioned, this book features five innovative workouts designed to burn fat and build muscle. You'll be doing fat-blasting aerobic workouts on Mondays, Wednesdays and Fridays. You can follow my aerobic routines or substitute any cardio activity of your choice (see pages 168 to 174 for some excellent options). Tuesdays and Thursdays are devoted to toning. Each of these workouts targets different muscle groups in different ways. On Saturdays, you'll be doing 60 minutes of any recreational activity of your choice, and Sunday is your day off. Once you get the hang of the program, you'll be able to whiz through your workouts without having to stop and consult the book to refresh your memory.

Over the next seven days, you'll be easing into Fidget-cize. Instead of doing one Fidget-cizer every hour—your ultimate goal—you'll be gradually adding these one-minute workouts into your day. Think of it as training yourself to get up out of your chair.

Week 1 is also the time to start reshaping your eating and lifestyle habits. Remember the Do's of Chapter 3? Eat your dinners as early as you can. On nights when an early dinner just isn't an option, simply keep your meal light and get back on track the next day.

Before getting started, find a blank notebook and make a few lists. First, I want you to think about all the reasons you've found it difficult to eat right or exercise in the past. Write them down, then brainstorm for solutions for each and every one. Next, write down your specific goals for the next four weeks. We already know that you want to lose 10 pounds. But would you also like to tone up your thighs? Tighten your abs? Reduce stress? Feel better about yourself? Finally, jot down at least five of your best characteristics—all the reasons that make you a great mother, friend, wife or husband, sister or brother. Think positive!

Over the next four weeks, use this notebook to record the details of your food intake and workouts. It takes only a few minutes, and it's a terrific way to identify hidden pitfalls and chart your progress.

Thought of the Week: Have a Positive Attitude!

For years, my friends and fans have asked me how I maintain such a positive outlook and always seem to be in a good mood. It's easy. I made the mental decision to be this way. Life is too short to waste time being negative. Happiness is a choice that is available to everyone. You just have to reach out and grab it!

There's some evidence that each of us is born with a happiness "set point." In other words, if you're a happy person, you'll always be a happy person; if you're a grouchy person . . . well, you get the picture. Despite temporary ups and downs, we eventually drift back to our base level of contentment. Fortunately, many experts believe that there are ways to change your happiness set point—in much the same way that you can boost your metabolism or lower your cholesterol. First step? Focus on the positive.

Maintaining a positive attitude has been linked to countless health benefits, including a lower risk of heart disease and a stronger immune system. Positive people are much more pleasant to be around. Other people look up to them, flock to them, turn to them for advice. They get job offers and raises, and become mentors for others. They're often the life of the party. I'm not promising a miracle. But I do promise that changing your attitude will change your life for the better. Enthusiasm is infectious, and the positive energy that you project into the world will come back to you tenfold.

For the next week, focus on how you react to situations. If one of your coworkers says something that hurts your feelings or another driver cuts you off, don't get angry or feel sorry for yourself. It's a waste of time and energy! *You* are the master of your emotions. Whenever steam starts coming out of my ears, I take three long, deep breaths and tell myself, "You are in control." Then I let go of the tension: I picture myself on a tropical island digging my toes into the warm sand. I relax my shoulders, soften my facial muscles and do a few neck rolls. If possible, I go for a walk—preferably outdoors.

While you're working on losing weight, I'll be feeding you with "Deniseologies"—positive affirmations aimed at reminding you of all your blessings and your potential for achievement. You *can* lose weight. You *can* exercise for 30 minutes. You *can* eat healthy meals. You can be anyone you want to be—I truly believe that! Now it's your turn.

I've learned through years of experience that recording your progress as you work toward a goal is one of the best ways to ensure success. So at the end of each week, we're going to have a personal progress report and "weigh in." By the end of your fourth week, your goal is to have lost 10 pounds—but you should also think in terms of inches. As you go through the program, you'll be building muscle, which weighs more than fat—so no matter what the scale says, you'll look thinner and firmer.

Before you get started, I want you to record your weight. After that, I want you to weigh yourself only once a week. Because you'll be losing fat and gaining muscle, the scale may not accurately reflect all the positive changes that you're making to your body. What's more, some women fluctuate by as much as four pounds due to fluid retention associated with their menstrual cycles; men may also gain or lose water depending on how much they're drinking and perspiring.

I've put a lot of people—both men and women—through this 28-day plan. The average weight loss was 10 pounds; some women lost closer to eight, while a few of the men lost as many as 14. Every body is different. But they all lost inches, especially around their waists. So I want you to take your measurements at the start and the end of the program, too. You also may want to have someone take a "before" photo of you in a pair of shorts or a swimsuit so you can really see the difference a little exercise and healthy eating makes.

WEIGH-IN: THE "BEFORE"

Complete the following chart on the morning of Day 1. After you've finished, don't look at these figures again until the four-week plan is done.

Day 1

Weight: _____ pounds
Measurements:

    1. Upper arm: Right: _____ inches
                                        Left: _____ inches
    2. Chest (across your bustline):   _____ inches
    3. Waistline: _____ inches
    4. Hips (around the widest point):   _____ inches
    5. Thighs (around the widest point):   _____ inches

Week 1 Shopping List

Healthy eating requires some preparation and planning! To make it easier on you, I've provided grocery lists at the beginning of each week. Be forewarned: The list for Week 1 is a bit longer than the rest. That's because you'll be buying all your condiments, canned goods and frozen foods for the next four weeks; only produce, meat and dairy products need to be purchased weekly.

Check the list carefully—it may include staples that you already have in your pantry.

I also recommend reading through all the daily menus before finalizing your list. There may be foods that you dislike or can't eat because of allergies. It's fine to substitute one meal for another or

> **Think positive and be optimistic— going through the motions can trigger the emotions!**

modify recipes slightly, trying to maintain a similar calorie count and balance of food groups. Since most of the recipes in the plan are designed for one person, if you're preparing meals for a family, now is the time to adjust the quantities on your shopping list accordingly.

PRODUCE

1 garlic bulb
1 14-ounce can flavored diced tomatoes
1 sweet potato, 4 inches long
1 Portobello mushroom
2 carrots
3 yellow onions
2 red onions
1 12-ounce jar roasted red peppers
3 1-pound packages frozen vegetables (one Birds Eye Oriental frozen veggie mix and two any variety)
1 bunch green onions
2 medium tomatoes
1 bunch endive
1 head broccoli
1 cup cauliflower
1 bag baby carrots
2 small zucchini
3 or 4 mushrooms
1 10-ounce bag baby spinach leaves
1 red, orange or yellow pepper
½ pound haricot verts
8 small red potatoes
½ pound sugar snap peas
1 10-ounce bag mixed greens

1 bunch celery
1 12-ounce jar fat-free bean dip
2 small containers prepared hummus
1 ginger root (keep this in the freezer)
1 10-ounce can black beans
1 9-ounce box raisins
1 9-ounce box Craisins
1 6-ounce bag of dried apricots
1-pound bag frozen sliced unsweetened peaches
2 fresh peaches
1 12- or 16-ounce container calcium-fortified orange juice
1 12-ounce bottle cranberry juice
3 Florida grapefruits
3 pints fresh or two 1-pound bags frozen, unsweetened mixed berries
3 bananas
2 oranges
1 cantaloupe
1 pear
3 Granny Smith apples
1 nectarine

2 20-ounce cans pineapple
chunks, in juice

DAIRY

1 quart skim milk
4 8-ounce containers low-fat
fruit-flavored yogurt
1 8-ounce container vanilla
yogurt
¼ pound sliced provolone
cheese
1 8-ounce container whipped
butter

MEAT/PROTEIN

¼ pound eye of round beef
1 jar natural chunky peanut
butter
¼ pound shaved smoked
turkey breast
1 package soy or veggie
burgers
1-pound package skinless,
boneless chicken breast
fillets

GRAINS

1 loaf multigrain bread
1 8-ounce bag egg noodles
6 whole-grain rolls, 3 inches
in diameter (freeze)
1 package whole-grain frozen
waffles
1 small piece focaccia bread
1 small box low-fat granola
or Grape-Nuts
1 12-ounce jar toasted wheat
bran
6 whole-wheat English muffins
6 bagels, 3.5 inches in diameter (freeze)
1 11.5-ounce box Multi-
Grain Cheerios
1 1-pound package 6-inch
whole-wheat pitas

2 lemons or bottle of lemon
juice
1 12-ounce bottle apple juice

1 16-ounce package shredded
light cheddar cheese
1 8-ounce package reduced-
fat feta cheese
1 6-ounce container grated
Parmesan cheese
1 12-ounce container low-fat
cottage cheese

1 8-ounce package frozen
crabmeat or imitation
crabmeat
6 eggs
1 4-ounce piece pork loin
1 4-ounce tuna steak
1 3-ounce can anchovies or
1 jar anchovy paste
(optional)

1 6-ounce package 3-inch
whole-grain pitas
1 13.5-ounce bag baked
tortilla chips
1 box Reduced Fat Triscuits
1-pound box rotini noodles
12 flour tortillas
12 corn tortillas, refrigerator-
style
1 18-ounce canister oatmeal
1 8-ounce box linguini
1 9-ounce box microwave
snack-size light popcorn
4-pack low-fat bran muffins
(freeze)
1-pound box phyllo dough
1 16-ounce box Fiber One
cereal

1 8-ounce box lasagna
   noodles
1 12-ounce box risotto

SPICES/CONDIMENTS/OIL

Worcestershire sauce
Plum sauce
Soy sauce
Vegetable spray
Olive oil
Red pepper flakes
1 small bottle "light" syrup
Raspberry mustard
1 jar salsa (mild, medium
   or hot)
Garlic powder
Fresh or dried rosemary
Vanilla
Onion powder
White pepper
1 small jar light mayonnaise
1 small bottle cocktail sauce
Pesto sauce
½ cup flour
1 large jar chunky pasta sauce
Citrus vinaigrette

MISCELLANEOUS

2 Denise Austin's Tasty Meal-
   to-Go bars, any flavor
1 pint fat-free sorbet, any
   flavor
1 9-ounce package light
   cheese tortellini
1 2.2-ounce bag slivered
   almonds
1 package raspberry herbal tea
1 package frozen cheese and
   potato pierogies
1 10.5-ounce can tomato or
   tomato basil soup
1 package green tea
1 box oat-cinnamon granola
   bars
3 boxes Cracker Jack

1 baguette—cut into 4-inch
   sections and freeze
1 14-ounce box calcium-
   fortified brown rice

Ginger teriyaki sauce
Paprika
Cinnamon
Lemon pepper marinade
Italian seasoning
1 3-ounce jar capers
1 8-ounce jar Dijonnaise
1 small jar green olives
1 12-ounce jar honey
Tabasco sauce
1 12-ounce jar fruit butter
1 12-ounce jar raspberry
   preserves
Old Bay seasoning
Tarragon vinegar
Dillweed
Cayenne pepper
White horseradish
Nutmeg
Salt
Pepper

1 box oat-fruit granola bars
1 box frozen fruit bars
1 package bouillabaisse mix
1 2.2-ounce bag cashew nuts
1 liter bottle flavored seltzer
   water
1 8-ounce container light
   whipped topping
1 10.5-ounce can minestrone
   soup
1 package biscotti
1 box instant vegetable broth
Sesame seeds
Oregano
1 package couscous
1 jar grainy mustard
Confectioners' sugar
Sugar

Day 1 MONDAY   *Ready, Set, Go!!!!!!*

DENISEOLOGY
*Become the most positive and enthusiastic person
you know. An optimistic outlook can awaken you to new
possibilities that often are buried by self-doubt and negativity.*

THE GAME PLAN

Today is the first day of a new, fit and healthy you! As you take your first aerobic steps, your first bites of good-for-you food, and try your first Fidget-cizers, remember that you'll be doing more than losing weight over the next four weeks. You'll be gaining energy, good health and, best of all, a better attitude. If you're feeling anxious about what lies ahead, simply focus on today and today only. Taking each day one step at a time will help keep you from feeling overwhelmed and appreciate the little successes you achieve along the way.

Here are a few more last-minute tips to help make this day, and the next 27, a little easier:

1. Get your food and exercise journal ready. You may want to carry it around with you so you can jot down notes as you go. Or keep it on your nightstand and record your successful day before bed—it's wonderful to dream about all you have accomplished and will accomplish!

2. If you can't keep up with a workout, slow down and do what you can. Moving counts, so just keep moving! The next time you exercise, you'll do a little more, and then a little more, and, before long, you won't remember way back when you couldn't finish a 30-minute workout.

3. Plan ahead! Schedule your workouts and treat them like an important meeting that you can't skip. The right mind-set will keep you from missing your daily dose of exercise.

4. Remember a simple equation: movement + healthy eating = new you. So move whenever you can, however you can. Follow my Fidget-cizers or make up your own. Focus on your day and when you find yourself sitting still, think about what you can do to keep your metabolism revved. Before long, it will be second nature to keep moving!

5. Avoid temptation of a different sort: Don't weigh yourself today, or any day except Monday mornings. You'll find weekly weigh-ins at the end of each week to help you chart your progress. Weighing yourself too soon always leads to frustration. This plan is designed for weight loss over 28 days, not one day. So no scales until next Monday!

Are you ready? Now get out there and move your way to a new lighter, healthier you!

- Start burning fat right off the bat! I want you to move, move, move for 30 minutes with any aerobic workout you love. If you prefer a set routine, go to pages 147 to 151 for a metabolism-boosting walk/jog interval workout. Walking is simply amazing exercise! Anyone can walk, anywhere, anytime. All you need is two legs and a pair of sturdy walking shoes. If you can't walk outside, you can do this workout on a treadmill.
- Practice Fidget-cize by doing squats (page 204) as you brush your teeth and tummy tucks (page 208) while you make meals or stop at a red light. Do as many Fidget-cizers as you can. Two is the absolute minimum.

DAILY TIP

Keep your feet happy! Good workout shoes will make any exercise much more enjoyable. A good fit and proper support are crucial for minimizing the stress on joints and avoiding injuries. Cushioned insoles help you go farther. Sweat-wicking, cushioned socks (not cotton) will help keep your feet comfy and blister-free.

All of the meal plans have "strive for five" in **bold** so you can see all the healthy fruits and veggies you are eating.

MEAL PLAN

Breakfast

MORNING GLORY SMOOTHIE

Combine the following in a blender:

4 ounces low-fat fruit-flavored yogurt
1/2 cup **fresh berries, sliced peaches** or **banana** or
    1/2 cup frozen, **unsweetened berries**
1/2 cup **orange juice**
1/3 cup toasted wheat bran

1 slice multigrain bread
1 teaspoon (one pat) whipped butter

Combine first four ingredients in blender until smooth. Enjoy with toasted bread and butter.

CALORIES	285
FAT	6.5 GRAMS
CALCIUM	253 MG
FIBER	12.2 GRAMS

Midmorning Snack

1 **pear**

CALORIES	60
FAT	0 GRAMS
CALCIUM	12 MG
FIBER	2.7 GRAMS

Lunch

PORTOBELLO MUSHROOM SANDWICH

1 large **Portobello mushroom**
1 teaspoon **garlic,** minced
1 teaspoon olive oil
1 splash Worcestershire sauce
1 dash **lemon juice**
1 whole-grain roll
1 piece **roasted red pepper**
1 slice provolone cheese
1 cup **strawberries**

Sauté mushroom in garlic, oil, Worcestershire sauce and lemon juice, about 5 minutes on each side. Cover and simmer for 10 minutes, or until tender. Serve on a whole-grain roll topped with roasted pepper and cheese. Enjoy the strawberries for dessert.

CALORIES	350
FAT	15 GRAMS
CALCIUM	282 MG
FIBER	4.2 GRAMS

Midafternoon Snack

One Denise Austin's Tasty Meal-to-Go bar, any flavor

CALORIES	220
FAT	5 GRAMS
CALCIUM	350 MG
FIBER	2 GRAMS

Dinner

GINGER BEEF VEGETABLE STIR-FRY

4 ounces thinly sliced eye of round beef
1 teaspoon olive oil
½ teaspoon grated ginger
1 cup frozen Oriental **vegetables**
½ cup dry egg noodles
1 tablespoon chunky peanut butter
1 tablespoon chopped **green onions**
1 dash red pepper flakes
1 teaspoon soy sauce

Sauté beef in a nonstick skillet with olive oil and grated ginger until pink in the middle, about 5 minutes. Remove meat from skillet and add frozen vegetables to the remaining liquid and sauté until crisp-tender, about four minutes. While meat is cooking, boil egg noodles according to package. Drain and mix with peanut butter, green onions, red pepper flakes and soy sauce. Top noodles with meat and vegetable mixture.

CALORIES	623
FAT	19 GRAMS
CALCIUM	73 MG
FIBER	6.4 GRAMS

TOTAL CALORIES FOR DAY 1	1,538
TOTAL FAT	45.5 GRAMS (26% OF CALORIES)
TOTAL CALCIUM	1,010 MG
TOTAL FIBER	25.3 GRAMS

Day 2 TUESDAY

DENISEOLOGY
Every person who has lost 10 pounds has had to lose that stubborn first pound as well, so be patient—and get busy!

THE GAME PLAN
• Today we'll be developing your muscles using more traditional weight-training moves like push-ups, squats and upright rows. If you're a beginner, practice doing the moves without weights until you feel comfortable. Once you're ready, do the moves again using light dumbbells (about 3 pounds each). If you've strength trained before, use enough weight to fatigue your target muscle by the final rep—but not so much that your form gets sloppy. Exhale as you lift and inhale as you lower. Ready? Turn to pages 154 to 166 for your toning routine.

• Go for four Fidget-cizers today. Pick from those pictured on pages 204 to 212 or make up your own.

DAILY TIP
Keep your mind on your muscles. When lifting weights, it's tempting to let your mind wander to the state of your current romantic relationship or that project you have due at the office next week. But if you focus your thoughts on the muscle that you're working, you'll get better results and really feel all the good that you're doing for your body.

MEAL PLAN

Breakfast

  2 whole-grain waffles with 2 tablespoons light syrup
  8 ounces skim milk

CALORIES	311
FAT	5.8 GRAMS
CALCIUM	456 MG
FIBER	2 GRAMS

Midmorning Snack

10 dried **apricot halves**

CALORIES	83
FAT	0.2 GRAM
CALCIUM	16 MG
FIBER	3.1 GRAMS

Lunch

TURKEY FOCACCIA SANDWICH

1 slice focaccia (3 inch by 3 inch by 1 inch)
1 sliced **tomato**
2 pieces **endive**
½ cup shaved smoked turkey breast
1 tablespoon raspberry mustard
1 medium **peach**

Make sandwich with first five ingredients. Have the peach for dessert or on the side.

CALORIES	343
FAT	7.6 GRAMS
CALCIUM	70 MG
FIBER	3.3 GRAMS

Midafternoon Snack

8 Reduced Fat Triscuits with 2 tablespoons light cream cheese

CALORIES	200
FAT	8 GRAMS
CALCIUM	40 MG
FIBER	4 GRAMS

Dinner

VEGETABLE FONDUE

1 tablespoon whipped butter
1 tablespoon flour
6 ounces skim milk
White pepper
Paprika
Onion powder
1 cup reduced-fat cheddar cheese
1 packet vegetable broth
2 cups assorted raw veggies cut in chunks (**broccoli, cauliflower, zucchini, mushrooms, baby carrots**)
½ cup lemon sorbet
1 cup fresh **berries**

Melt butter and stir in flour and milk. Stir until smooth and thickened. Flavor with pepper, paprika and onion powder. Add cheddar cheese and stir until melted. Boil 8 ounces water; add vegetable broth and vegetables to heat them slightly. Using fondue forks, dip vegetables in cheese fondue and enjoy. Serve sorbet and berries for a refreshing dessert.

CALORIES	634
FAT	29 GRAMS
CALCIUM	1,088 MG
FIBER	14.7 GRAMS

TOTAL CALORIES FOR DAY 2	1,571
TOTAL FAT	51 GRAMS (29% OF CALORIES)
TOTAL CALCIUM	1,630 MG
TOTAL FIBER	27.1 GRAMS

Day 3 WEDNESDAY

DENISEOLOGY
Food isn't the enemy; sitting still is.

THE GAME PLAN
- Another beautiful morning! Smile as you take two minutes to think happy thoughts about the day ahead and the great job that you're doing.
- Time for another aerobic blast! As on Day 1, choose your favorite 30-minute cardio workout. Or, do my Fat-Burning Blast workout on pages 168 to 176. This workout will keep you moving for 30 minutes with a mixture of heart-pumping and strength-building exercises. Get ready to sweat!
- Aim to Fidget-cize at least six times today. Flip to pages 204 to 212 for a how-to.

DAILY TIP
If you're sore from these new exercise routines, don't give up! Instead, keep moving. Research shows that the best remedy for exercise-induced soreness is getting right back on the horse. By stretching or going for a walk, you'll pump nutrients to your muscles to speed healing. Exercise = feeling better faster. Why not give it a go?

MEAL PLAN

Breakfast

> 1 small, low-fat bran muffin topped with 1 teaspoon whipped butter
> 6 ounces skim milk

CALORIES	289
FAT	6.2 GRAMS
CALCIUM	292 MG
FIBER	4 GRAMS

Midmorning Snack

> 1 cup **mixed berries,** fresh or frozen
> 1 biscotti

CALORIES	110
FAT	1.5 GRAMS
CALCIUM	27 MG
FIBER	8.4 GRAMS

Lunch

FETA-SPINACH VEGGIE BURGER

> Vegetable spray
> 1 soy-based vegetable burger
> ½ cup fresh **spinach leaves**
> 2 ounces reduced-fat feta cheese
> 2 tablespoons **salsa**
> 1 whole-grain roll
> ½ **Florida grapefruit**

If not using the microwave, coat a nonstick skillet with vegetable spray and lightly sauté veggie burger. Top with spinach, feta and salsa. Serve on whole-grain roll. Have the grapefruit in wedges on the side or for dessert.

CALORIES	413
FAT	16 GRAMS
CALCIUM	432 MG
FIBER	9 GRAMS

Midafternoon Snack

> 1 box Cracker Jack

CALORIES	150
FAT	2.5 GRAMS
CALCIUM	0 MG
FIBER	1 GRAM

Dinner

ROSEMARY CHICKEN

½ chicken breast
1 teaspoon olive oil
Garlic powder or half a **garlic** clove, minced
¼ teaspoon dried rosemary or 1 teaspoon fresh rosemary
1 cup **sugar snap peas**
4 small **red potatoes**

Preheat oven to 350 degrees. Brush chicken breast with olive oil and sprinkle with garlic powder or fresh garlic and rosemary. Cover with foil and bake until cooked through (about 20 minutes). Steam 1 cup sugar snap peas until crisp-tender. Boil potatoes and season with olive oil, garlic powder and rosemary. Enjoy!

CALORIES	511
FAT	13.7 GRAMS
CALCIUM	94 MG
FIBER	7 GRAMS

TOTAL CALORIES FOR DAY 3	1,473
TOTAL FAT	39.9 GRAMS (24% OF CALORIES)
TOTAL CALCIUM	845 MG
TOTAL FIBER	29.4 GRAMS

Day 4 THURSDAY

DENISEOLOGY
You can go from fat to flab-free at any age!

THE GAME PLAN

• Today is the day to start building muscle! My yoga and Pilates-inspired resistance exercises on pages 179 to 193 can truly change the shape of your body. This is a softer form of strength training; no weights are required. You'll love the results—strong, flexible muscles; long, lean limbs; better balance and beautiful posture. This is also your half hour to reconnect your mind and your muscles. Start by turning off your phone and TV. Eliminate as many distractions as you can. Because these exercises focus on balance and deep breathing, they help draw your consciousness inward to nurture your soul and provide more mental clarity than, say, a fast-paced workout like interval training. I do moves like these several times a week to keep my body and my spirit balanced. I know you'll grow to love, and crave, these mind-body exercises as much as I do.

• Fidget-cize! I call them my *invisible* exercises! Let's go for eight today. Pretty soon you'll be doing them subconsciously! Turn to page 212 and pick from my list, or make up your own.

DAILY TIP

Standing up straight can make you look 10 pounds thinner—and 10 years younger! So practice keeping your abdominals pulled in and your shoulders back. Pretend you're holding a winning lottery ticket between your shoulder blades, or that there is a string at the top of your head that's pulling you toward the ceiling. The sky's the limit!

MEAL PLAN

Breakfast

YOGURT PARFAIT

   4 ounces low-fat yogurt
   ½ cup fresh or frozen **blueberries**
   1 tablespoon Grape-Nuts or granola

In a tall glass, layer half the yogurt, berries and cereal. Repeat.
Enjoy!

CALORIES	323
FAT	3 GRAMS
CALCIUM	355 MG
FIBER	4.4 GRAMS

Midmorning Snack

   1 oat-cinnamon granola bar

CALORIES	100
FAT	3 GRAMS
CALCIUM	0 MG
FIBER	1.5 GRAMS

Lunch

CRAB SANDWICH

   4 ounces crabmeat or imitation crab
   1 tablespoon light mayonnaise
   1 tablespoon cocktail sauce
   1 whole-wheat English muffin
   2 **lettuce** leaves
   1 **apple**

Combine the first three ingredients. Toast English muffin and
top with crab salad and lettuce. Enjoy an apple for dessert.

CALORIES	503
FAT	6.8 GRAMS
CALCIUM	191 MG
FIBER	16.1 GRAMS

Midafternoon Snack

1 tablespoon natural chunky peanut butter on
1 **celery stalk**

CALORIES	100
FAT	8 GRAMS
CALCIUM	6.5 MG
FIBER	2.15 GRAMS

Dinner

TORTELLINI WITH SIDE SALAD

3 ounces light cheese tortellini
2 cups **mixed greens**
2 tablespoons **Craisins**
2 tablespoons citrus vinaigrette
½ cup chunky pasta sauce

Cook tortellini according to package. Toss mixed greens with Craisins and vinaigrette. Heat sauce and pour over pasta.

CALORIES	500
FAT	10.4 GRAMS
CALCIUM	301 MG
FIBER	6 GRAMS

TOTAL CALORIES FOR DAY 4	1,526
TOTAL FAT	31.2 GRAMS (18% OF CALORIES)
TOTAL CALCIUM	853 MG
TOTAL FIBER	30.15 GRAMS

Day 5 FRIDAY

DENISEOLOGY
You are as you think, so why not think healthy, fit and happy?

THE GAME PLAN
- Time for another 30 minutes of fat-blasting exercise! Today's workout is circuit training—a mix of short bursts of aerobic exercise and muscle-building weight moves. Two workouts in one! The goal is to keep your heart rate elevated, so move quickly from one move to the next. For example: You'll start by jumping rope for three minutes, then do one set of triceps dips; from there, you'll move into an ab-toning yoga pose for one minute, then get your heart rate going again with two minutes of squat jumps. If you opt to do your favorite aerobic workout instead, try my *Sizzler* or *Fat-Burning Blast* videos for a real aerobic charge.
- Today I want you to try 10 Fidget-cizers. See pages 204 to 212 and get moving!

DAILY TIP
Tone your arms while you shop for food! You have to lift those bags anyway, so why not build your biceps simultaneously? Curl your arms up and down as you carry your groceries to the car and into your house. Canned goods make excellent weights!

MEAL PLAN

Breakfast

PEANUT BUTTER AND JELLY SANDWICH

    1 tablespoon natural chunky peanut butter
    1 tablespoon honey, preserves or fruit spread
    2 slices multigrain bread
    1 5-inch **banana**

Make sandwich with first three ingredients. Enjoy with banana.

CALORIES	387
FAT	11 GRAMS
CALCIUM	50 MG
FIBER	8.7 GRAMS

Midmorning Snack

    1 oat-cinnamon granola bar

CALORIES	100
FAT	3 GRAMS
CALCIUM	0 MG
FIBER	1.5 GRAMS

Lunch

SOUP AND PIEROGIES

    3 cheese-potato pierogies
    1/2 cup raw **spinach**
    1 cup **tomato** or **tomato basil soup**
    1 **nectarine**

Prepare pierogies according to package. Add spinach leaves to soup and heat. Enjoy a juicy nectarine for dessert.

CALORIES	315
FAT	5.2 GRAMS
CALCIUM	100 MG
FIBER	8.2 GRAMS

Midafternoon Snack

8 ounces low-fat yogurt
½ cup **berries**
1 tablespoon preserves
¼ cup low-fat granola

Top yogurt with berries, preserves and granola for a refreshing afternoon pick-me-up!

CALORIES 379
FAT 4.8 GRAMS
CALCIUM 399 MG
FIBER 3.4 GRAMS

Dinner

TUNA TERIYAKI

1 **sweet potato**
4-ounce tuna steak
2 tablespoons ginger teriyaki sauce
1 cup **haricot verts**
1 teaspoon olive oil
1 teaspoon **garlic**, minced
Orange juice
Cinnamon

Bake sweet potato. Brush both sides of tuna steak with teriyaki sauce. Grill or broil until cooked through, about 5 minutes per side. Sauté haricot verts with olive oil and garlic for about 5 minutes. Serve potato with a splash of orange juice and a sprinkle of cinnamon.

CALORIES 380
FAT 6 GRAMS
CALCIUM 125 MG
FIBER 3.4 GRAMS

TOTAL CALORIES FOR DAY 5 1,561
TOTAL FAT 33 GRAMS (19% OF CALORIES)
TOTAL CALCIUM 674 MG
TOTAL FIBER 25.2 GRAMS

Day 6 SATURDAY

> ## DENISEOLOGY
> *If you rest, you rust!*

THE GAME PLAN

• Smile—it's Play Day! Today, I want you to do one hour of recreational physical activity, preferably outside so you can soak up the fresh air and sun. Go in-line skating, play tennis, ride a bike, swim or explore a new hiking trail with your friends or your kids. On Saturdays, my husband Jeff and I like to take the kids to the playground. We shoot hoops, hang from the monkey bars, play catch and run around. When the kids are on the swings, I do my own mini-workout while keeping a watchful eye on them. Park benches are perfect for doing triceps dips and step-ups. Or I stand on a curb and do calf raises. If the weather is bad, go ice-skating, bowling or mall walking. Exercise doesn't have to mean solitary, boring or tedious. It can include anything from swing dancing to gardening to simply lacing up comfy shoes and hitting the road. Even an energetic game of Ping-Pong counts! Have a great day playing.

• I know it's Play Day, but don't forget to Fidget-cize! Today's goal is 12. Turn to pages 204 to 212 for suggestions.

DAILY TIP

When you exercise as a family, you get to spend quality time together as you teach your kids the importance of working out and a healthy lifestyle. Everyone wins!

MEAL PLAN

Breakfast

VEGETABLE OMELETTE

2 eggs
Vegetable cooking spray
½ cup Oriental or frozen **vegetables**
1 tablespoon grated Parmesan cheese
1 slice whole-grain bread

1 teaspoon butter
1 teaspoon preserves

Lightly whisk eggs. Coat omelette pan with vegetable spray and add eggs. Allow egg mixture to travel down sides of the pan to create a fluffy egg base. Add veggies and cheese. Cook for about 2 minutes, or until egg is cooked through. Serve with toasted bread topped with butter and preserves.

CALORIES	346
FAT	17 GRAMS
CALCIUM	179 MG
FIBER	6.3 GRAMS

Midmorning Snack

1 cup raspberry herbal tea with a splash of **cranberry juice**

CALORIES	20
FAT	0 GRAMS
CALCIUM	0 MG
FIBER	0 GRAMS

Lunch

COTTAGE CHEESE PARFAIT

¾ cup low-fat cottage cheese or part-skim ricotta
½ cup **pineapple chunks**
½ cup **mixed berries**
1 tablespoon slivered almonds
1 multigrain bagel

Layer cottage cheese, pineapple, berries and almonds. Repeat. Serve with toasted bagel.

CALORIES	516
FAT	13 GRAMS
CALCIUM	308 MG
FIBER	4.6 GRAMS

Midafternoon Snack

¼ cup **hummus** with ½ cup **baby carrots**

CALORIES	136
FAT	5 GRAMS
CALCIUM	50 MG
FIBER	5.3 GRAMS

Dinner

ROASTED PORK LOIN

4-ounce piece pork loin
¼ cup **yellow onion**, chopped
½ cup pasteurized **apple juice** or **cider**
½ cup **carrot** chunks
1 peeled **Granny Smith apple**, cut into wedges
1 4-inch **potato**, cut into chunks
Rosemary
Onion powder
Pepper
1 cup **broccoli**
Lemon juice

Preheat oven to 350 degrees. In a pan, brown pork loin with onion and apple juice. Transfer to a baking pan. Add carrots, apple and potato. Season meat with dash of rosemary, onion powder and pepper. Cover with foil and bake 30 minutes or until no longer pink in the middle. Steam broccoli and douse with lemon juice.

CALORIES	489
FAT	13.5 GRAMS
CALCIUM	116 MG
FIBER	11 GRAMS

TOTAL CALORIES FOR DAY 6	1,507
TOTAL FAT	48.5 GRAMS (29% OF CALORIES)
TOTAL CALCIUM	653 MG
TOTAL FIBER	27.2 GRAMS

Day 7 SUNDAY

DENISEOLOGY

*When you approach an activity with confidence,
you will perform beyond your expectations.*

THE GAME PLAN

• You did it! You made it through your first week. If you're tired, take the day off—you deserve it. Even better, keep up the good work by continuing to move . . . nothing too strenuous! On Sundays, I like to try something new or treat myself to a full hour of yoga or meditation. I also use this day to get organized for the week ahead. It's a good time to stock up on groceries and do a little prep work to make meals during the week as quick and easy as possible. Often, I'll cook a chicken or make a big vegetable lasagna that I can divide into separate portions and then store in the freezer. Or I'll cut up some fresh veggies, such as carrots, celery, cucumbers and red peppers, so I don't have to spend time chopping on busy weekday nights. I also take five minutes to plan my workouts for the coming week, then write them into my calendar—a terrific way to make sure they actually happen!

• Today you're going to add two more Fidget-cizers (see pages 204 to 212) for a total of 14. At this point, you should be doing one about every hour or so from the moment you rise and shine until bedtime. I do *at least* this many every day—in my opinion, it's one of the best defenses against middle-age spread!

DAILY TIP

Hydrate, hydrate, hydrate! Water is our lifeblood. Even if you're taking a rest day, keep drinking. Water is important both when you exercise and when you don't. Waiting until you're thirsty is a big mistake—by that time, you'll already be dehydrated. So run to the kitchen and pour yourself a big glass of H_2O. Cheers!

MEAL PLAN

Breakfast

> 1 cup Multi-Grain Cheerios
> ¼ cup **raisins**
> 8 ounces skim milk

CALORIES	248
FAT	1.9 GRAMS
CALCIUM	342 MG
FIBER	4.36 GRAMS

Midmorning Snack

> 8 Reduced Fat Triscuits
> 1 cup herbal tea

CALORIES	130
FAT	3 GRAMS
CALCIUM	0 MG
FIBER	4 GRAMS

Lunch

SPINACH-TOMATO-FETA MELT

> 1 whole-grain pita
> 1 teaspoon olive oil
> ½ cup **spinach leaves**
> 1 sliced **tomato**
> ¼ cup crumbled feta cheese
> 1 **orange**

Brush pita with olive oil and top with spinach, tomato and feta. Broil until cheese melts. Cut the orange in wedges and serve on the side.

CALORIES	453
FAT	19 GRAMS
CALCIUM	376 MG
FIBER	7.7 GRAMS

Midafternoon Snack

13 baked tortilla chips
¼ cup fat-free **bean dip**
2 tablespoons **salsa**

CALORIES	170
FAT	1 GRAM
CALCIUM	40 MG
FIBER	4.4 GRAMS

Dinner

CHICKEN CACCIATORE

Vegetable spray
½ skinless, boneless chicken breast (4 ounces)
½ cup **chunky pasta sauce**
½ cup dry rotini noodles
2 cups **romaine lettuce**
½ **orange, yellow** or **red pepper**
½ cup **pineapple chunks**
1 tablespoon grated Parmesan cheese
2 tablespoons vinaigrette

Preheat oven to 350 degrees. Spray baking dish with vegetable spray. Place chicken breast in dish and top with pasta sauce. Cover with foil and bake for 20 minutes, or until chicken is cooked through. While chicken is cooking, boil noodles according to package. Make salad with remaining five ingredients. Place cooked chicken mixture on bed of noodles.

CALORIES	546
FAT	10 GRAMS
CALCIUM	192 MG
FIBER	4.9 GRAMS

TOTAL CALORIES FOR DAY 7	1,547
TOTAL FAT	34.9 GRAMS (20% OF CALORIES)
TOTAL CALCIUM	950 MG
TOTAL FIBER	25.36 GRAMS

Week 1—Weekly Weigh-In

So how did your first week go? I hope it went great, and that you're already feeling the benefits of your healthy new eating and exercise habits. If you experienced some muscle soreness, remember that this is normal and will go away soon. Drink lots of water and keep moving and stretching for better circulation and to minimize the aches.

Now is the time to check your progress. Step on the scale first thing tomorrow morning (Monday—Day 8) before you eat or drink anything, preferably wearing nothing but your "birthday suit."

Record Week 1 Weight

Day 8: _____ pounds

I hope you've seen some improvement. My goal for you is to lose about two and a half pounds per week. If you're not on target, don't worry: Just stick with my eating and exercise program, and your body will respond soon. Also, you may have been eating too late at night. I want you to really try to eat dinner as early as possible so you can burn off some of those calories before going to sleep. If you have difficulty putting a curfew on your kitchen, try my favorite trick: Brush your teeth right after eating so you feel finished for the evening; plus, food doesn't taste as good after you have toothpaste in your mouth.

In addition to losing a little weight, you should start to see some tightening and toning of your muscles. And you're probably feeling more energetic, too! By now, eating right and exercising should have become part of your daily routine. If you've missed a workout or you've cheated and pigged out, remember that the first week is the hardest. So forge ahead and do better in Week 2.

Make a vow to yourself that you are going to stay dedicated. You'll be so much happier. It'll be worth it! A little success breeds enthusiasm and more motivation to keep going. Step by step, you're on your way to a goal. You're going to lose those 10 pounds, and lose them for good. You're going to feel better than ever!

5 | Week Two

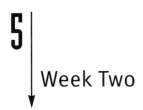

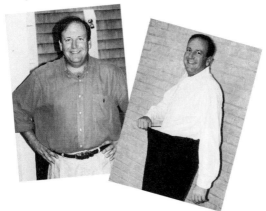

Tom *stuck with my program for five months and lost 50 pounds total— 14 in the first month. He also lost four inches in his waistline and his cholesterol dropped from 200 to 136. "I feel great, thanks to Denise."*

WEEK AT A GLANCE

MONDAY: Cardio—Walk/jog intervals (30 minutes)
Mind-Body-Spirit Routine (5 minutes)

TUESDAY: Toning—Weight training (30 minutes)

WEDNESDAY: Cardio—Fat-Burning Blast with light weights
(30 minutes)
Mind-Body-Spirit Routine (5 minutes)

THURSDAY: Toning—Yoga and Pilates Method (30 minutes)

FRIDAY: Cardio—Triple cardio mix with muscle-toning circuit
(30 minutes)
Mind-Body-Spirit Routine (5 minutes)

SATURDAY: Play Day (60 minutes)

SUNDAY: Rejuvenation Day

You should be proud of yourself! Week 1 is done, and you're already making progress. You are starting to feel thinner, firmer and more energetic; perhaps you're even beginning to look forward to your workouts. And no doubt that Fidget-cize is becoming a habit! But success doesn't mean that you can slow down.

Just the opposite, in fact. This week, you're going to up the ante by picking up the pace during your aerobic workouts and adding new muscle-building moves. Are you ready to *really* ignite your metabolism? Onward!

Thought of the Week: Learn to Like Yourself!

Fate didn't grant me a fit body, a loving husband and a successful career. Sure, I've been lucky. But I've also worked hard to get where I am. There were plenty of times that I wanted to give up, when all that effort didn't seem worth it. But I persevered and didn't take "No" for an answer—and it paid off.

> "No one can make you feel inferior without your consent."
>
> **—ELEANOR ROOSEVELT**

My big break came in 1984, when I became the fitness consultant for NBC's *Today* show. In those days, none of the morning news shows covered fitness, but I had a hunch that it could be a hit. After more than 30 phone calls to a *Today* show producer, I finally landed a meeting with him. As I walked into his office, my heart was pounding. I sat in his office trying to talk to him as he casually practiced his swing with a baseball bat. But I got the job. After my first appearance on the show, the network received more than 10,000 letters. I had proved myself!

The first step to liking yourself is to realize that no one's perfect. Everyone has fat days. Bad-hair days. Days when you change outfits a hundred times and still don't like what you see. It's just a part of life. You can't expect a complete attitude adjustment overnight. But you can start taking baby steps toward a better self-image. You are worthy—convince yourself, and others will think it, too!

How do you turn negatives into positives? Stop beating yourself up about what you *aren't* and focus on what you *are*. Ban phrases like "jelly belly" and "thunder thighs" from your vocabulary. Body-image experts tell us that even when you don't vocalize your discontent, other people can sense your insecurities. Your wide frown and droopy slouch sends out "I don't feel good about myself" signals. Big mistake!

Take some time this week to remind yourself that you're an incredible, unique individual with so much to offer. Applaud what is special about you. Don't think, "Fat." Think, "Smart, funny, interesting, motivated, giving, beautiful."

If you feel those old doubts and insecurities start to resurface, engage in a little positive self-talk. List your five best attributes in your head or out loud, or write them down in a journal. If you're still doubtful, ask someone whom you trust to help you with your list. What does he or she think your best qualities are? Review the list every night before you go to bed, or carry it with you so you can pull it out whenever those self-critical thoughts pop into your head.

Don't let self-doubt become a self-fulfilling prophecy. Make a conscious effort to stop putting yourself down, both in your own mind and your conversations with others. When you enter a room, do it with confidence—hold your chin up, pull your shoulders back and smile. A great, big wide smile!

Be positive, be proud! Each day you practice your new habits will make you healthier, happier, stronger and more energetic. Confidence in your abilities will do more to help you keep that weight off forever than any diet ever could. You are a unique and rare individual—the one and only you! Celebrate who you are and what you're working to become. Your radiance will spread to those around you.

Week 2 Shopping List

PRODUCE

1 ripe mango
3 baking potatoes
1 8-ounce can mandarin
  oranges
1 8-ounce can black beans
1 pound red grapes
1 nectarine
1 pound asparagus
1 pint berries, any variety
1 small eggplant

1 peach
1 pear
1 tangerine
1 4-pack container natural
  applesauce
1 cantaloupe
1 bunch fresh basil
1 small head broccoli
2 mushrooms
1 Granny Smith apple

DAIRY

1 ounce fresh mozzarella
  cheese
¼ pound sliced, smoked
  Gouda cheese
1 8-ounce package shredded
  part-skim mozzarella cheese

1 8-ounce container light
  cream cheese
1 8-ounce container vanilla
  yogurt
1 small container low-fat sour
  cream

MEAT/PROTEIN

1 10-ounce package baby
  shrimp
6 large shrimp
1 pound ground turkey breast

2 3-ounce cans salmon
1 1-pound package turkey
  breast fillets
1 4-ounce filet mignon

Day 8 MONDAY

DENISEOLOGY
Posture speaks volumes; make sure yours says "Confidence!"

THE GAME PLAN

- Today you're going to get your metabolism moving with 30 minutes of fat-blasting aerobics. Do my walk/jog interval workout (pages 147 to 151), or pick another favorite. If you decide to be your own boss, don't forget to vary your workout. If you walked on Saturday, try biking today. Or step up the metabolism-boosting quality of your workout by increasing your intensity. The harder you work, the more calories you burn!
- Use Fidget-cize (pages 204 to 212) to enhance your posture. Elongate your spine as you sit or stand. Get up and stretch. Standing tall becomes you!

DAILY TIP

To get more out of your walking workout, pay attention to your posture. Hold your chest up and shoulders back. Pull your abdominals in tight and don't arch your back. Your feet should be about hip-width apart, with your toes pointing straight ahead. Plant your heel on the ground and roll through to the ball of your foot and push off of your toes. Keep your arms bent at 90-degree angles and your elbows in close to your sides. Really pump those arms! The more muscles you use, the more calories you'll burn. To boost your bottom line, squeeze your buttocks when you walk (like I do) . . . because if you don't squeeze it, no one else will!

MEAL PLAN

Breakfast

SCRAMBLED EGG BURRITO

2 eggs
1 tablespoon skim milk
Vegetable spray
2 tablespoons **salsa**

1 white or whole-wheat tortilla
1 half **cantaloupe**

Scramble eggs with milk. Coat a nonstick pan with vegetable spray and cook eggs until done. Spoon eggs and salsa into tortilla. Enjoy with fresh cantaloupe.

CALORIES	335
FAT	13.7 GRAMS
CALCIUM	135 MG
FIBER	2 GRAMS

Midmorning Snack

1 **Florida grapefruit,** peeled

CALORIES	78
FAT	0.2 GRAM
CALCIUM	28 MG
FIBER	12.0 GRAMS

Lunch

VEGGIE SANDWICH WITH SOUP

1 whole-grain roll
Olive oil
1 **tomato,** sliced
¼ cup fresh **basil leaves**
1 ounce fresh mozzarella
½ cup **broccoli florets**
1 cup **minestrone soup**
1 **peach**

Cut roll in half and brush with olive oil. Broil until lightly browned. Top each side with tomato, basil and mozzarella. Add broccoli florets to soup and heat. Top off your meal with a peach.

CALORIES	380
FAT	12.4 GRAMS
CALCIUM	255 MG
FIBER	13.3 GRAMS

Midafternoon Snack

    1 small, low-fat bran muffin

CALORIES	200
FAT	3 GRAMS
CALCIUM	66 MG
FIBER	3.9 GRAMS

Dinner

SHRIMP AND VEGGIE KABOBS

    ¼ cup brown rice
    3 large shrimp
    2 **mushrooms**
    ½ cup **red onion**, cut in chunks
    ½ small **zucchini**, cut in chunks
    ½ **red, yellow,** or **green pepper** cut in wedges
    2 tablespoons lemon pepper vinaigrette
    ½ ripe **mango** cut into strips

Cook brown rice according to package. While rice is cooking, skewer shrimp, mushrooms, onion, zucchini and peppers. Brush with vinaigrette. Broil or grill until shrimp turns pink. Serve over rice. Enjoy mango—a cooling, tropical dessert.

CALORIES	569
FAT	12 GRAMS
CALCIUM	117 MG
FIBER	7.2 GRAMS

TOTAL CALORIES FOR DAY 8	1,562
TOTAL FAT	41.3 GRAMS (24% OF CALORIES)
TOTAL CALCIUM	601 MG
TOTAL FIBER	38.4 GRAMS

Day 9 TUESDAY

DENISEOLOGY

The fastest way to reshape your body is by lifting weights.
The weights you lift are worth their weight in gold!

THE GAME PLAN

• Today, ignite your metabolism with my weight-training routine on pages 154 to 166. Pay attention to form as you do each move. You want to move your target muscles through a full range of motion. For example, if you're doing biceps curls, lift the weight all the way up, then lower it *all* the way down to starting position.

• You're beginning to see the beauty of "Fidget-cize." You not only burn calories, you keep those muscles loose—no stiffness or trouble getting up! Next time you're on the phone telling your friend how great you feel, do a wall sit (page 207). Terrific for the thighs!

DAILY TIP

You can boost your fiber intake by eating whole fruits and vegetables instead of drinking juice. Juicing breaks down the fiber content in fruit. So slice an apple or peel a grapefruit to add extra fiber—and flavor—to your day.

MEAL PLAN

Breakfast

BAKED APPLE

1 **Granny Smith apple**
¼ cup **orange juice**
⅓ cup dry oats
¼ cup toasted wheat bran
2 teaspoons butter, melted
1 tablespoon brown sugar
Cinnamon
4 ounces low-fat vanilla yogurt

Preheat oven to 350 degrees. Peel and slice apple and place in a baking dish. Pour orange juice on top. In a separate bowl mix together oats, wheat bran, butter, brown sugar and cinnamon. Sprinkle oat mixture over apple. Bake for 15 to 20 minutes. Top with yogurt. What a great way to start your day!

CALORIES	469
FAT	11.5 GRAMS
CALCIUM	198 MG
FIBER	8.9 GRAMS

Midmorning Snack

1 cup herbal tea with a splash of **orange juice**

CALORIES	20
FAT	0 GRAMS
CALCIUM	0 MG
FIBER	0 GRAMS

Lunch

BOUILLABAISSE

1 serving **bouillabaisse** (about 1½ cups prepared)
½ package (5 ounces) frozen baby shrimp, thawed
1 whole-grain roll
1 teaspoon whipped butter
½ cup **pineapple chunks**

Prepare bouillabaisse according to package. Add baby shrimp and cook 2 to 3 minutes, or until shrimp are pink. Serve with roll and butter. For dessert: pineapple!

CALORIES	446
FAT	11.3 GRAMS
CALCIUM	155 MG
FIBER	4.7 GRAMS

Midafternoon Snack

¾ cup Multi-Grain Cheerios with 4 ounces skim milk

CALORIES	122
FAT	0.75 GRAM
CALCIUM	190 MG
FIBER	2.25 GRAMS

Dinner

FILET MIGNON

4-ounce filet mignon
1 clove **garlic**, chopped
Italian seasoning
Worcestershire sauce
1 cup **broccoli**
2 teaspoons olive oil
1 teaspoon sesame seeds
1 baked **potato**
Olive oil
Garlic powder

Marinate filet in garlic, Italian seasoning and Worcestershire sauce. Broil until pink in the middle. Sauté broccoli in olive oil and top with sesame seeds. Cut baked potato into wedges, brush lightly with olive oil and sprinkle with garlic powder. A hearty meal for a hard worker!

CALORIES	511
FAT	20.6 GRAMS
CALCIUM	106 MG
FIBER	9.6 GRAMS

TOTAL CALORIES FOR DAY 9	1,568
TOTAL FAT	44 GRAMS (25% OF CALORIES)
TOTAL CALCIUM	649 MG
TOTAL FIBER	25.5 GRAMS

Day 10 WEDNESDAY

THE GAME PLAN

- Rise and shine! Don't just smile—laugh out loud!
- OK, I bet you're *really* beginning to feel the benefits of regular exercise. You feel stronger, leaner, livelier. You're sleeping well. Your skin positively glows. Well, keep moving! Today's dose: 30 minutes of fat-blasting aerobics. Do my Fat-Burning Blast on pages 168 to 176 or any heart-pumping activity of your choice.
- Fidget-cize! If you haven't tried one of the mini-workouts pictured on pages 204 to 212, today's the day!

DAILY TIP

Whenever possible, exercise outdoors so you can soak up the fresh air and sun (don't forget your SPFs!). You'll enjoy your workout more, and it'll do wonders for your outlook on life!

MEAL PLAN

Breakfast

PEACH SMOOTHIE

> 4 ounces lemon yogurt
> 4 ounces skim milk
> ½ cup frozen or fresh sliced **peaches**
> ½ cup **orange juice**
> ¼ cup toasted wheat bran
> 3 ice cubes
> 1 biscotti

I like to use my Osterizer blender to blend the first six ingredients for a nutritious breakfast drink. Serve with biscotti.

CALORIES	398
FAT	4.4 GRAMS
CALCIUM	333 MG
FIBER	7.5 GRAMS

Midmorning Snack

1 cup **raspberries**, fresh or frozen

CALORIES	60
FAT	0 GRAMS
CALCIUM	0 MG
FIBER	8.4 GRAMS

Lunch

TURKEY BURGER

¼ pound ground turkey breast or 1 prepackaged
turkey burger
Soy, teriyaki or Worcestershire sauce
Garlic powder
Oregano
1 whole-grain bun
2 slices **roasted red pepper**
1 tablespoon country mustard
1 cup **red grapes**

Combine ground turkey, sauce, garlic powder and oregano, then shape into a patty. Grill or broil and serve on whole-grain bun with roasted red pepper and mustard. Enjoy grapes for dessert!

CALORIES	380
FAT	14 GRAMS
CALCIUM	77 MG
FIBER	2.9 GRAMS

Midafternoon Snack

Make this midafternoon snack a double dose! Walk to your local frozen yogurt shop—you'll be getting double the benefit!

1 small, or kiddie-size, cone of frozen yogurt, any flavor

CALORIES	100
FAT	0.8 GRAM
CALCIUM	112 MG
FIBER	0 GRAMS

Dinner

VEGETABLE QUESADILLAS

1 teaspoon olive oil
1 clove **garlic**, minced
¼ cup **onion**, chopped
¼ cup **mushrooms**, chopped
¼ cup **zucchini**, chopped
¼ cup **broccoli**, chopped
¼ cup **cauliflower**, chopped
½ cup canned, chopped **tomatoes**
2 flour tortillas
2 ounces Gouda cheese (about two thin slices)

Heat olive oil and sauté garlic until translucent. Add onion, mushrooms, zucchini, broccoli, cauliflower and tomatoes. Cook until tender. Divide vegetable mixture onto two tortillas and top each with an ounce of Gouda. Place under broiler briefly to melt cheese. *Olé!*

CALORIES	576
FAT	27 GRAMS
CALCIUM	622 MG
FIBER	6.4 GRAMS

TOTAL CALORIES FOR DAY 10	1,514
TOTAL FAT	46.2 GRAMS
TOTAL CALCIUM	1,144 MG
TOTAL FIBER	25.2 GRAMS

Day 11 THURSDAY

DENISEOLOGY
*Eating right isn't about willpower;
it's about changing those bad habits!*

THE GAME PLAN

• It's time to work and lengthen those muscles! Turn to pages 179 to 193 for my yoga and Pilates-based resistance routine. Focus on tightening your abdominal muscles as you do each one. Your body will move into proper alignment, and you'll become more aware of how all your muscles work together as a unit. Before long, you'll find yourself walking and moving with greater ease and grace—more like a dancer! Your posture should improve, too. Exercise doesn't just help us lose weight, it helps create a healthy, happy body from head to toe.

• Fidget-cize! You can Fidget-cize right now by doing a few leg lifts or tapping your toes as you read. If you're moving, it counts!

DAILY TIP

Don't forget to breathe—all day long and especially during your workouts. Deep breathing will help keep your mind in the moment so you get more out of your exercises. Inhale through your nose to deliver energy-boosting oxygen to your muscles. Exhale slowly through your mouth to release stress and tension from your entire body. You should be able to hear the sound of your breath as oxygen enters and leaves your body. Imagine that you're "breathing in" energy and "exhaling out" stress.

MEAL PLAN

Breakfast

¾ cup Multi-Grain Cheerios
¾ cup low-fat granola
8 ounces skim milk
1 banana

CALORIES	396
FAT	3.5 GRAMS
CALCIUM	359 MG
FIBER	6.4 GRAMS

Midmorning Snack

1 pear

CALORIES	60
FAT	0 GRAMS
CALCIUM	12 MG
FIBER	2.7 GRAMS

Lunch

SALMON SANDWICH

1 3-ounce can salmon, drained
3 tablespoons Dijonnaise
1 whole-wheat English muffin, toasted
1 **tomato**, sliced
2 **celery** stalks, cut into small pieces
1 **tangerine**

Combine salmon and Dijonnaise. Divide evenly between two English muffin halves and top with tomato slices. Serve with celery. End your meal with a refreshing tangerine!

CALORIES	362
FAT	9.8 GRAMS
CALCIUM	328 MG
FIBER	8.3 GRAMS

Midafternoon Snack

1 package snack-size microwave light popcorn

CALORIES	155
FAT	3.7 GRAMS
CALCIUM	3 MG
FIBER	8.1 GRAMS

Dinner

PASTA PUTTANESCA

1 ounce linguini (about the size of a quarter in diameter)
¾ cup **chunky pasta sauce**
1 tablespoon capers
1 finely chopped anchovy or 1 teaspoon anchovy paste
    (optional)
Red pepper flakes
2 cups **mixed greens**
4 ounces **mandarin oranges** (about ½ cup)
2 tablespoons citrus vinaigrette

Prepare linguini according to package. Heat pasta sauce, adding capers, anchovy and red pepper flakes to taste. Top cooked linguini with sauce. Toss greens with oranges and vinaigrette.

CALORIES	573
FAT	9.8 GRAMS
CALCIUM	328 MG
FIBER	5.4 GRAMS

TOTAL CALORIES FOR DAY 11	1,546
TOTAL FAT	26.8 GRAMS (16% OF CALORIES)
TOTAL CALCIUM	1030 MG
TOTAL FIBER	30.9 GRAMS

Day 12 FRIDAY

> ## DENISEOLOGY
> *When you finish a workout, you don't simply feel better—*
> *you feel better about yourself.*

GAME PLAN

• Friday is fat-blasting day! Turn to pages 195 to 202 for your Circuit Training workout. Or do 30 minutes of your favorite aerobic activity. Remember: To burn maximum calories, you want to keep changing your routine. Create your own calorie-burning circuit workout! If you're jogging, run up a hill, do 15 push-ups, sprint to the nearest tree, then jump up and touch a branch. Try to engage as many movement patterns and muscle fibers as possible.

• Today you're going to add another Fidget-cizer, for a grand total of 16—one for every waking hour. Start now: Stand up, take a deep breath and stretch! That's it!

DAILY TIP

Watch TV from the floor. It's the best seat in the house—especially when it comes to getting toned! So as soon as you hear the words "stay tuned," start moving. During each commercial break, do one 15-rep set of one of the following exercises: leg lifts, push-ups, triceps dips and crunches. Who ever said TV was a waste of time?

MEAL PLAN

Breakfast

> 1 whole-grain bagel
> ¼ cup low-fat cottage cheese
> ¼ cup **pineapple chunks**
> Cinnamon
> 1 cup herbal tea

Split bagel in half and top each side with cottage cheese, pineapple chunks and a sprinkle of cinnamon. Enjoy with a flavorful cup of tea!

CALORIES	351
FAT	2.45 GRAMS
CALCIUM	99 MG
FIBER	4.2 GRAMS

Midmorning Snack

1 oat-cinnamon granola bar

CALORIES	100
FAT	3 GRAMS
CALCIUM	0 MG
FIBER	1.5 GRAMS

Lunch

BLACK BEAN QUESADILLAS

2 corn tortillas
⅔ cup **black beans**
1 tablespoon **salsa**
1 tablespoon **green onions**
1 tablespoon light sour cream
2 tablespoons light cheddar cheese, grated
1 **nectarine**

Slightly warm tortillas in microwave or oven. Place warm tortillas on broiler pan and top each one with black beans, salsa, onions, light sour cream and cheese. Broil until cheese melts. Dessert is a juicy nectarine.

CALORIES	490
FAT	15 GRAMS
CALCIUM	666 MG
FIBER	14.75 GRAMS

Midafternoon Snack

½ **Florida grapefruit**

CALORIES	40
FAT	0 GRAMS
CALCIUM	0 MG
FIBER	6.0 GRAMS

Dinner

CHICKEN PARMESAN

1 teaspoon olive oil
1/2 chicken breast (4 ounces)
1/2 cup **chunky pasta sauce**
2 tablespoons Parmesan cheese
1/3 cup couscous
1 1/2 cups **asparagus**
1 teaspoon sesame oil
1/2 teaspoon grated ginger
1/2 clove **garlic**, minced

Preheat oven to 350 degrees. Add olive oil to nonstick skillet and lightly brown chicken. Transfer to baking dish and cover with pasta sauce and cheese. Bake for 20 minutes, or until chicken is cooked through. While chicken is baking, prepare couscous according to package and sauté asparagus in sesame oil with ginger and garlic until crisp-tender. Top couscous with chicken; serve with asparagus. Delicious!

CALORIES	537
FAT	19 GRAMS
CALCIUM	270 MG
FIBER	7 GRAMS

TOTAL CALORIES FOR DAY 12	1,518
TOTAL FAT	39 GRAMS (23% OF CALORIES)
TOTAL CALCIUM	1,069 MG
TOTAL FIBER	34.45 GRAMS

Day 13 SATURDAY

DENISEOLOGY

If you can walk or bike, don't drive. Finding a more challenging way to get to your destination is not only a great, practical way to burn calories—it's fun!

THE GAME PLAN

- It's Saturday! Time to get out there and play. Do anything you want. Try trail running or mountain biking. Play 18 holes of golf (walk the course—don't ride!). And whatever happened to badminton? If it rains, briskly walk a mall or dig out the Ping-Pong paddles. Just be sure to keep going for at least 60 minutes. If you'll be exercising for more than an hour, bring water and a healthy snack. Enjoy the day!
- I know it's Play Day, but don't forget to Fidget-cize! You've done great all week—keep the fire alive!

DAILY TIP

Dance your dinner off! Whether you're out on a Saturday night or staying home, turn on your favorite tunes. The beat will keep you moving your feet, not to mention burning off those calories!

MEAL PLAN

Breakfast

FRIED EGG SANDWICH

1 egg
Vegetable spray
Tabasco sauce
2 slices multigrain bread, toasted
¼ **cantaloupe**

Fry egg in vegetable spray. Add a dash of Tabasco for pizzazz! Serve on multigrain toast. Enjoy with fresh cantaloupe.

CALORIES	254
FAT	7.6 GRAMS

CALCIUM   79 MG
FIBER   6.8 GRAMS

Midmorning Snack

    1 cup fresh **mixed berries** with 2 tablespoons low-fat
       whipped topping

CALORIES   65
FAT   1 GRAM
CALCIUM   0 MG
FIBER   3.4 GRAMS

Lunch

SPINACH SALAD

    2 cups baby **spinach leaves**
    ½ cup baby shrimp (remaining ½ package)
    2 tablespoons cashews
    2 tablespoons citrus vinaigrette
    1 whole-grain roll
    1 4-ounce container **natural applesauce**

Toss together spinach, shrimp, cashews and vinaigrette. Serve
with roll. Satisfy your sweet tooth with applesauce!

CALORIES   466
FAT   12.9 GRAMS
CALCIUM   224 MG
FIBER   6.5 GRAMS

Midafternoon Snack

    1 small, low-fat bran muffin

CALORIES   200
FAT   3 GRAMS
CALCIUM   66 MG
FIBER   3.9 GRAMS

Dinner

VEGGIE-STUFFED POTATO

1 5-inch baked **potato**
2 tablespoons light sour cream
Onion powder
1 cup **mixed vegetables: broccoli, carrots, cauliflower,**
    and **mushrooms**
1 teaspoon olive oil
2 ounces smoked Gouda cheese (about two slices)

Scoop out filling of baked potato and mix with sour cream and onion powder. Return filling to potato skin. Sauté vegetables in olive oil until crisp-tender. Cover potato with vegetables and top with cheese. Broil until cheese melts.

CALORIES	543
FAT	22.1 GRAMS
CALCIUM	506 MG
FIBER	8.4 GRAMS

TOTAL CALORIES FOR DAY 13	1,528
TOTAL FAT	46.6 GRAMS (27% OF CALORIES)
TOTAL CALCIUM	875 MG
TOTAL FIBER	29 GRAMS

Day 14 SUNDAY

DENISEOLOGY
Instead of thinking of your body as the enemy,
think of it as your best friend.

GAME PLAN:
• Congratulations! You made it through the second week. That wasn't so bad, was it? Today's your day to do anything your heart desires. Lounge around the house, run errands or take a leisurely walk. Even better, pamper yourself. On my free days, I like to place votive candles all around my bathroom and relax in a warm bath filled with lavender oil. Sometimes to be more productive, you need to be less productive. You've earned it!

• I know it's your day off, but try to keep up with your Fidgetcize. Every little bit helps.

DAILY TIP
Plant an indoor herb garden. Fresh herbs bring so much fragrance and flavor to each meal! Add savory parsley, chives, basil and sage to salads, pastas, poultry—you name it. Or snip a few pretty sprigs and place them in a water-filled vase on your windowsill. The scent will delight you throughout the day and inspire you to put extra care into your meals.

MEAL PLAN

Breakfast

RICE PUDDING

⅔ cup cooked brown rice
½ cup skim milk
2 tablespoons toasted wheat bran
1 egg, beaten
2 tablespoons **raisins**
1 tablespoon sugar, honey or syrup

Combine above ingredients in a saucepan and heat for about 5 to 7 minutes (about 2 minutes in a microwave).

CALORIES	387
FAT	5.6 GRAMS
CALCIUM	197 MG
FIBER	5.48 GRAMS

Midmorning Snack

10 dried **apricot halves**

CALORIES	83
FAT	0 GRAMS
CALCIUM	16 MG
FIBER	3.1 GRAMS

Lunch

EGGPLANT PARMESAN

¼ **eggplant**, peeled and sliced into ¼-inch thick slices (if you don't like eggplant, substitute a 6-inch **zucchini**)
2 teaspoons olive oil
½ cup **chunky pasta sauce**
2 tablespoons shredded part-skim mozzarella cheese
2 tablespoons grated Parmesan cheese
1 whole-grain roll
Garlic powder

Preheat oven to 350 degrees. Pat eggplant slices with paper towels to remove extra moisture and brush both sides of each using 1 teaspoon olive oil. Broil or grill for 5 minutes. Place eggplant slices in a small baking dish and cover with ¼ cup sauce and 1 tablespoon each of mozzarella and Parmesan. Repeat with remaining eggplant, sauce and cheese. Bake for 15 minutes. Serve with garlic toast: Cut whole-grain roll in half and brush with remaining olive oil and garlic powder, then broil lightly.

CALORIES	447
FAT	20.5 GRAMS
CALCIUM	278 MG
FIBER	4 GRAMS

Midafternoon Snack

Florida grapefruit, peeled

CALORIES	80
FAT	0 GRAMS
CALCIUM	0 MG
FIBER	12.0 GRAMS

Dinner

HONEY MUSTARD TURKEY BREAST FILLET

2 tablespoons water
4 ounces skinless turkey breast fillet
1 tablespoon honey
1 tablespoon grainy mustard
Lemon juice
3 small **potatoes,** boiled
Skim milk
Garlic powder
2 tablespoons light cream cheese
1 cup **mixed vegetables,** steamed
Vinaigrette

Preheat oven to 350 degrees. Pour water into baking dish and add turkey. Mix together honey, mustard and splash of lemon juice. Spoon over turkey. Cover with foil and bake for 20 to 25 minutes. Mash boiled potatoes with skim milk, garlic and cream cheese. Top steamed vegetables with a splash of vinaigrette. *Bon appétit!*

CALORIES	554
FAT	6.4 GRAMS
CALCIUM	198 MG
FIBER	10.14 GRAMS

TOTAL CALORIES FOR DAY 14	1,551
TOTAL FAT	32.5 GRAMS (19% OF CALORIES)
TOTAL CALCIUM	689 MG
TOTAL FIBER	34.7 GRAMS

Week 2—Weekly Weigh-In

You've made it to the halfway point! How do you feel? I hope great. . . . Your body is starting to get stronger, transforming you into a fit and healthy person.

Now is the time to check your progress. Step on the scale first thing tomorrow morning (Monday—Day 15) before you eat or drink anything, preferably wearing only your "birthday suit."

Record Week 2 Weight

Day 15: _____ pounds

Hopefully you've seen some progress. Have you lost about five pounds since Day 1? If you have, you're on target. Even if you've lost only three pounds, you should be proud of yourself, because the fact is—you're improving! Remember, we are working off and losing true BODY FAT—shedding excess fat, not just water weight! So even though the numbers may be small, the benefit is big!

Be patient—results will come if you stay with the program. I know at times you'll be tempted to give up or cheat on your diet . . . so go ahead and give yourself a "treat" once a week. Maybe pick a Friday or Saturday night. It's OK to do this once a week, but no more, because multiple "cheat" days take you off-track and keep you from the success I know you want and I know that you can achieve.

If you stumble once in a while, put it behind you, clean your slate and keep going onward and upward. Focus on your progress—YOU CAN DO IT! Remember, each day you have a chance to succeed, even if only in a very small way. Each small success contributes to the next small success. Each is a separate building block toward your overall goal of positive habits.

Make an oath with yourself. Write your promise down to help you accomplish your goal. GO FOR IT—you'll look and feel better than ever!

6

Week Three

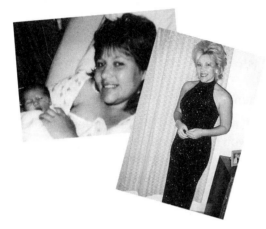

Wendy lost 45 pounds after having her baby by following my plan for four months.

WEEK AT A GLANCE

MONDAY: Cardio—Walk/jog intervals (30 minutes)
Mind-Body-Spirit Routine (5 minutes)

TUESDAY: Toning—Weight training (30 minutes)

WEDNESDAY: Cardio—Fat-Burning Blast with light weights
(30 minutes)
Mind-Body-Spirit Routine (5 minutes)

THURSDAY: Toning—Yoga and Pilates Method (30 minutes)

FRIDAY: Cardio—Triple cardio mix with muscle-toning circuit
(30 minutes)
Mind-Body-Spirit Routine (5 minutes)

SATURDAY: Play Day (60 minutes)

SUNDAY: Rejuvenation Day

You're over the hump! In Week 3, you'll *really* begin to see some results. More endurance and stamina. Stronger muscles. Looser clothes. Don't let up now—the end's in sight! So keep up your healthy eating habits. Really give your workouts your all. And give yourself a pep talk. You're not going to give up. You want this. You can do it! Believe it, and it will be so!

Thought of the Week: Stop and Smell the Roses

I know what you're thinking: "Denise just said to exercise nonstop, and now she tells me to take time out for flowers?"

Let me explain. A good life should be busy, organized and full of purpose. But sometimes life's most pleasurable moments and opportunities get squeezed out of the agenda. Suppose you are off on a brisk walk when you see a beautiful lilac bush just bursting into bloom. You could walk right by so as not to break your stride—but it can be just as rewarding to stop a moment to enjoy the wonderful scent of those perfect, tiny lavender petals. When you start up again, you will begin to see, sniff and feel the wonder of everything around you. As your body breathes in freshness, your mind and spirit are aired out as well. By momentarily putting aside your immediate agenda, you have gained something greater—a reawakened appreciation for the world that will fuel all of your other activities throughout the day.

Breaking away from your goals and routines, however briefly, can have myriad benefits for your well-being and your health. Did you know that hives, pimples, insomnia, teeth grinding, indigestion and even *weight gain* are often a result of stress? More seriously, some experts believe that stress may be a contributing factor to heart disease. Instead of fretting about the busy day to come, while you exercise, focus on clearing your head and making room for new experiences. Naturally we can't just snap our fingers to forget responsibilities and personal problems, but we can try to put anxieties aside for a few minutes to rest our minds and put things into proper perspective. Your step will seem lighter and your workout shorter when you focus on pleasant, positive thoughts. Best of all, you will be countering the stress that is so harmful to your health.

When you finish your walk or workout, stop again. Allow yourself a moment of pure peace. Remember how important your health is to your whole family and how great it feels to be cranking through this program. Then smile. Kiss a kid. Pat a dog. Smell a rose. There's always time for the best things in life. And they're free!

Week 3 Shopping List

PRODUCE

1 red pepper
2 pints mixed berries or 1 bag
    frozen berries
1 bunch green onions
3 Florida grapefruits
4 apples
1 cantaloupe
1 tomato
½ cup baby carrots
1 head endive
1 cup red grapes
2 bananas
1 bag mixed greens
1 peach or ½ cup frozen
    sliced peaches

1 potato
4 oranges
½ pound snow peas
3-pound wedge of water-
    melon
1 pear
10-ounce bag baby spinach
1 small eggplant
1 small zucchini
2 ears of corn
4 bananas
1 small head broccoli
1 bunch parsley
1 nectarine

DAIRY

4 8-ounce containers yogurt
    (1 vanilla, 3 fruit-flavored)
¼ pound Muenster cheese
3 slices reduced-fat Alpine
    Lace cheese

1 quart skim milk
1 8-ounce container part-
    skim ricotta
¼ pound Asiago cheese

MEAT/PROTEIN

1 6.5-ounce can clams
2 3-ounce cans water-packed
    tuna
1 4-ounce chicken breast,
    turkey breast fillet or piece
    of tofu
1 6-ounce can salmon
1 package black bean burgers

¾ pound shaved ham or
    smoked turkey breast
1 4-ounce piece eye of round
    beef or sirloin steak
1 4-ounce piece orange
    roughy, cod, sole or
    flounder
6 eggs

Day 15 Monday

THE GAME PLAN

- Start Week 3 with a wide smile. You know that you're making progress and you feel better already.
- Time to burn fat with 30 minutes of aerobics! Do my walk/run interval workout on pages 147 to 151, or stick with your favorite cardiovascular activity. If it's a rainy day, follow along with my Lifetime TV show. You're doing great—keep up the good work!
- Don't forget to Fidget-cize—make sure you move once every hour. If you're stuck in a long business meeting, try isometrics (page 212)—no one has to know that you're tightening your tush during work hours.

DAILY TIP

Try a change of scenery! If you've been running, biking or in-line skating in your neighborhood, experiment with a different route or try a new locale altogether. Drive to a nearby park or to a friend's house and experience a whole new world. With so much more to look at and appreciate, you'll spend less time focusing on how many minutes are left on your workout.

MEAL PLAN

Breakfast

FRENCH TOAST

> 1 egg
> ¼ cup skim milk
> 2 slices multigrain bread
> Vegetable spray
> Cinnamon
> Confectioners' sugar
> ½ cup **mixed berries**, sliced

In a small bowl, beat egg with milk, add bread and soak thoroughly. Coat nonstick pan with vegetable spray, add bread and cook until browned on each side. Sprinkle with cinnamon, sugar and berries.

CALORIES	339.5
FAT	15 GRAMS
CALCIUM	174.5 MG
FIBER	7.7 GRAMS

Midmorning Snack

1 5-inch **banana**

CALORIES	105
FAT	0.5 GRAM
CALCIUM	7 MG
FIBER	2.7 GRAMS

Lunch

TORTELLINI SALAD

⅓ package light cheese tortellini
1 cup frozen **mixed vegetables**
2 tablespoons light vinaigrette
½ cup **baby carrots**
1 4-ounce container **natural applesauce**

Cook tortellini and toss with vegetables. Add vinaigrette and chill. Add carrots and enjoy! Have applesauce for dessert.

CALORIES	491
FAT	9.5 GRAMS
CALCIUM	215 MG
FIBER	7.3 GRAMS

Midafternoon Snack

8 ounces low-fat yogurt with ¼ cup Fiber One

CALORIES	255
FAT	3.1 GRAMS
CALCIUM	334 MG
FIBER	6.5 GRAMS

Dinner

FAJITAS

> 4-ounce skinless, boneless chicken breast, 4-ounce turkey
>   breast fillet or 4-ounce piece extra-firm tofu
> 2 tablespoons bottled fajita sauce
> 1 teaspoon olive oil
> ½ **green, red** and **yellow pepper**, julienned
> ½ **red** or **yellow onion**, thinly sliced
> 2 flour, whole wheat, or corn tortillas
> 2 tablespoons **salsa**

Cut chicken, turkey or tofu into finger-size strips. Marinate in fajita sauce. Grill or broil until cooked through—about 5 to 7 minutes. In a separate pan, heat olive oil. Add peppers and onion. Cook until crisp-tender. Warm tortillas in oven or microwave. Divide meat and veggies between tortillas. Top with salsa.

CALORIES	347
FAT	10.3 GRAMS
CALCIUM	124 MG
FIBER	1.9 GRAMS

TOTAL CALORIES FOR DAY 15	1,537.5
TOTAL FAT	38.4 GRAMS (22% OF TOTAL CALORIES)
TOTAL CALCIUM	854.5 MG
TOTAL FIBER	26.4 GRAMS

Day 16 TUESDAY

DENISEOLOGY
If you recline, you decline. If you sit, you quit. If you don't use it, you'll lose it. And we need all the metabolism-boosting muscle we can get!

THE GAME PLAN
• Turn to pages 154 to 166 for your weight-training workout. Today, think "good form," good technique and body alignment—quality over quantity. Focus on using slow, controlled movements and working your muscles through a full range of motion. If you can complete all reps easily, it's time to add weight. Your goal is to get stronger, so keep your muscles challenged!

• Move, move, move! Make sure you're Fidget-cizing every hour on the hour.

DAILY TIP
If you have a busy morning—your kids need to be at school early or you have a breakfast meeting at work—split your workout in two. Do half in the morning and half in the late afternoon or evening. It may not feel like it, but you're doing your muscles just as much good!

MEAL PLAN

Breakfast

FRUIT AND YOGURT SUNDAE
1 cup **mixed berries** and **cantaloupe**
4 ounces vanilla yogurt
1 teaspoon honey
Splash **lemon juice**
1 tablespoon slivered almonds
1 slice multigrain bread, toasted
1 teaspoon whipped butter

Top fruit with yogurt, honey, lemon juice and almonds. Serve with toast and butter.

CALORIES	374
FAT	14.2 GRAMS
CALCIUM	244 MG
FIBER	6.2 GRAMS

Midmorning Snack

1 cup raspberry herbal tea with ¼ cup **cranberry juice**

CALORIES	20
FAT	0 GRAMS
CALCIUM	0 MG
FIBER	0 GRAMS

Lunch

VEGGIE SANDWICH

2 slices multigrain bread
1 slice Muenster cheese
¼ cup **hummus**
½ **tomato**, sliced
2 slices **red onion**
1 **Granny Smith apple**

Top one bread slice with cheese and one with hummus, then top both with tomato and onion. Put halves together and enjoy. Munch on an apple for dessert—and to keep the doctor away!

CALORIES	462
FAT	16.6 GRAMS
CALCIUM	311 MG
FIBER	12.1 GRAMS

Midafternoon Snack

1 stalk **celery** with 1 tablespoon natural chunky peanut butter

CALORIES	97
FAT	8 GRAMS
CALCIUM	20 MG
FIBER	2.7 GRAMS

Dinner

PASTA WITH CLAM SAUCE

2 cups **mixed greens**
2 tablespoons **Craisins**
4 ounces **mandarin oranges**
2 tablespoons light vinaigrette
1 ounce dry linguini (about a quarter inch in diameter)
½ cup canned clams
Dash cayenne pepper
¾ cup **chunky pasta sauce**

Toss together greens, Craisins, oranges and vinaigrette. Set aside. Cook pasta. Mix together clams, pepper and sauce. Pour over pasta. *Mangia!*

CALORIES	634
FAT	9 GRAMS
CALCIUM	193 MG
FIBER	6.9 GRAMS

TOTAL CALORIES FOR DAY 16	1,587
TOTAL FAT	47.8 GRAMS (27% OF TOTAL CALORIES)
TOTAL CALCIUM	775 MG
TOTAL FIBER	27.9 GRAMS

Day 17 WEDNESDAY

THE GAME PLAN

• Eliminate flab and tension with my 30-minute Fat-Burning Blast workout (pages 168 to 176) or any aerobic workout of your choice.

• Today, focus on doing stress-reducing Fidget-cizers: neck stretches, upper-back stretches and lower-back stress relievers (pages 204 to 212).

DAILY TIP

Try something you're not that good at. My husband, Jeff, comes from a tennis-playing family; he played on the pro circuit and his sister, Tracy Austin, is a U.S. Open champion. Even though many of my shots land in the net, I get out and hit the ball with him on a regular basis. With tennis, I exercise muscles that I don't normally use. I really feel it the next day! So be willing to try an activity or sport that isn't your best; your body will thank you, and who knows? You may discover an unknown skill.

MEAL PLAN

Breakfast

PEACHY BREAKFAST BLAST

½ cup Fiber One cereal
¾ cup Multi-Grain Cheerios
6 ounces skim milk
½ cup fresh or frozen sliced **peaches**

Combine the above and greet the day with a smile!

CALORIES	214.5
FAT	1.75 GRAMS
CALCIUM	300.5 MG
FIBER	16.1 GRAMS

Midmorning Snack

2 slices reduced-fat Alpine Lace Swiss cheese and 1 **apple**

CALORIES	244
FAT	6 GRAMS
CALCIUM	440 MG
FIBER	3.6 GRAMS

Lunch

TUNA NIÇOISE

3-ounce can water-packed tuna, drained
2 tablespoons light vinaigrette
1 tablespoon capers
5 sliced green olives
1 cup **endive**
1 whole-grain bagel
1 tablespoon fruit butter
1 cup **red grapes**

Toss tuna with vinaigrette, capers, olives and serve on a bed of endive. Serve with toasted bagel topped with fruit butter. For dessert: grapes!

CALORIES	434
FAT	7.6 GRAMS
CALCIUM	71 GRAMS
FIBER	3.6 GRAMS

Midafternoon Snack

Make your afternoon snack today a double dose! Walk to your local ice cream shop—you'll be getting double the benefit!

½ cup lemon sorbet

CALORIES	120
FAT	0 GRAMS
CALCIUM	0 MG
FIBER	0 GRAMS

Dinner

BLACK BEAN BURGER

1 **black bean burger**
1 whole-grain roll
1 slice **roasted red pepper**
½ cup fresh **baby spinach**

Broil, grill or microwave burger. Place on roll and top with roasted pepper and spinach.

CALORIES	456
FAT	7.5 GRAMS
CALCIUM	335 MG
FIBER	5.5 GRAMS

TOTAL CALORIES FOR DAY 17	1,468
TOTAL FAT	22.8 GRAMS (14% OF TOTAL CALORIES)
TOTAL CALCIUM	1,146.5 MG
TOTAL FIBER	28.8 GRAMS

Day 18 THURSDAY

DENISEOLOGY
Remind yourself why you're working so hard:
for your health, for your body, for your mind, for you!
God gave us one body—take good care of it!

THE GAME PLAN

- Time to shape and sculpt your metabolism-boosting muscles. Go to pages 179 to 193 for your yoga and Pilates-based toning workout.
- Keep Fidget-cizing! Next time you're in line at a grocery store or filling up your gas tank, do calf raises while you wait. Every movement counts!

DAILY TIP

When doing abdominal exercises, place your fingers on the area you're trying to work. Go slowly—don't use a jerking motion. Press your belly button toward your spine. And breathe! Exhale as you tighten your tummy and inhale as you release. The result? Abs-olutely fabulous!

MEAL PLAN

Breakfast

BREAKFAST BURRITO

½ cup part-skim ricotta
1 teaspoon sugar
Splash vanilla
1 flour tortilla
1 teaspoon strawberry preserves
½ cup sliced **strawberries**

Blend ricotta, sugar and vanilla. Warm tortilla and spread with preserves. Spoon in ricotta mixture and top with strawberries. What a festive way to start your day!

CALORIES	263
FAT	6 GRAMS

CALCIUM	204 MG
FIBER	1.3 GRAMS

Midmorning Snack

1 oat-cinnamon granola bar and 1 cup raspberry herbal tea

CALORIES	100
FAT	3 GRAMS
CALCIUM	0 MG
FIBER	1.5 GRAMS

Lunch

SOUP AND SANDWICH

1 whole-wheat pita bread
3 ounces shaved maple ham or smoked turkey
1 thin slice Muenster cheese
1 cup **minestrone soup**
1 **pear**

On bread, make sandwich with ham or turkey and cheese. Heat soup and enjoy! The finale: a pear.

CALORIES	365
FAT	8.7 GRAMS
CALCIUM	304 MG
FIBER	4.8 GRAMS

Midafternoon Snack

⅓ cup **hummus** on 8 Reduced Fat Triscuits

CALORIES	261.5
FAT	9.5 GRAMS
CALCIUM	38.4 MG
FIBER	7.9 GRAMS

Dinner

BEEF STIR-FRY

4 ounces eye of round or sirloin steak
2 tablespoons plus a splash ginger teriyaki sauce
2 teaspoons olive oil
1 teaspoon **garlic,** minced
1 **green onion,** chopped
1½ cups frozen **Oriental vegetables**
⅔ cup cooked brown rice

Marinate beef in teriyaki sauce. Heat 1 teaspoon olive oil, garlic and onion in nonstick pan. Add beef. Cook until pink in the middle. Remove from heat and place in separate dish. Set aside. Using same pan, add remaining olive oil and vegetables and stir-fry until crisp-tender. Add beef and a splash of teriyaki sauce and mix. Serve over brown rice.

CALORIES	529
FAT	10.5 GRAMS
CALCIUM	90 MG
FIBER	12.7 GRAMS

TOTAL CALORIES FOR DAY 18	1,518.5
TOTAL FAT	37.7 GRAMS (22% OF TOTAL CALORIES)
TOTAL CALCIUM	636.4 MG
TOTAL FIBER	28.2 GRAMS

Day 19 FRIDAY

THE GAME PLAN

- I love fat-burning Fridays! Follow along with me for 30 minutes of Circuit Training (pages 195 to 202), or pick your own aerobic workout.
- Do every Fidget-cizer you've learned—and get ready for a fun-filled weekend!

DAILY TIP

Feeling like you just won't make it through today's workout? Slip into Lycra. It's hard to believe, but "compression" workout clothing can up your endurance and power, according to a five-year study conducted at Pennsylvania State University.

MEAL PLAN

Breakfast

½ **cantaloupe**
½ cup low-fat cottage cheese
1 slice multigrain bread
1 teaspoon whipped butter

Top cantaloupe with cottage cheese. Toast bread and serve with butter.

CALORIES	245
FAT	6.8 GRAMS
CALCIUM	105 MG
FIBER	2.8 GRAMS

Midmorning Snack

4 ounces fruit-flavored yogurt with ¼ cup **raspberries**

CALORIES	170
FAT	2 GRAMS
CALCIUM	150 MG
FIBER	4.2 GRAMS

Lunch

TOMATO-CHEESE BAGUETTE

1 4-inch-long baguette
1 teaspoon olive oil
1 **tomato,** sliced
½ cup sliced **basil**
¼ cup Asiago cheese, shredded
1 **nectarine**

Cut baguette in half and brush each half with ½ teaspoon olive oil. Broil until slightly browned. Top each half with tomato, basil and cheese. Broil until cheese melts. Follow it up with a nectarine!

CALORIES	522
FAT	22.7 GRAMS
CALCIUM	747 MG
FIBER	3.2 GRAMS

Midafternoon Snack

½ cup low-fat **bean dip** with 1 serving baked tortilla chips (13 chips)

CALORIES	217
FAT	1.6 GRAMS
CALCIUM	44 MG
FIBER	9.4 GRAMS

Dinner
My favorite meal—a reminder of my runs along the Potomac River!

CRAB-SALMON PATTIES

1 5-inch-long **potato**, washed and thinly sliced
1 teaspoon olive oil
Paprika
6-ounce can salmon
4-ounce package crabmeat or imitation crab
2 tablespoons bread crumbs
½ **red pepper**, finely chopped
2 tablespoons Dijonnaise
Dash onion powder
Dash Old Bay seasoning
Vegetable spray
1 cup **snow peas**
1 teaspoon white horseradish
1 tablespoon mustard or Dijonnaise
Splash soy sauce

Preheat oven to 350 degrees. Brush potato slices with olive oil and sprinkle with paprika. Bake for 30 minutes or until tender. While potato bakes, combine salmon and crab. Add bread crumbs, red pepper, Dijonnaise, onion powder and Old Bay seasoning. Form two patties. Wrap one patty in plastic wrap and save for tomorrow's lunch. Coat nonstick skillet with vegetable spray. Cook patty until brown on one side, then flip and brown the other. While patty is cooking, steam snow peas. Combine horseradish and mustard. Serve patty with horseradish-mustard sauce, potato and snow peas splashed with soy sauce.

CALORIES	399
FAT	9.2 GRAMS
CALCIUM	223 MG
FIBER	8.1 GRAMS

TOTAL CALORIES FOR DAY 19	1,553
TOTAL FAT	42.3 GRAMS (25% OF TOTAL CALORIES)
TOTAL CALCIUM	1,269 MG
TOTAL FIBER	27.7 GRAMS

Day 20 SATURDAY

THE GAME PLAN

- Play Day! All the work that you've been doing during the last three weeks will really pay off today. You'll have the energy and endurance to truly enjoy 60 minutes of your favorite sport or activity.
- Today, pick Fidget-cizers that make you feel strong. Triceps dips, squats, kicks and punches will build muscle, burn calories and leave you feeling empowered. See pages 204 to 212 for ideas.

DAILY TIP

Think before you drink. You consume a lot of extra calories by sipping soda or juice instead of water. Club soda, seltzer and decaffeinated iced tea are all good choices—as long as they're not filled with sugar. Caffeinated beverages give you an instant jolt, but as diuretics, they ultimately rob your body of water . . . and there's not much worse for energy levels than dehydration.

MEAL PLAN

Breakfast

EGG CHEESE BAKE

2 eggs
Splash skim milk
Salt and pepper to taste
¼ cup shredded light cheddar cheese
1 6-ounce glass calcium-fortified **orange juice**
2 slices whole-grain bread, toasted
1 tablespoon fruit butter

Preheat oven to 350 degrees. Beat eggs with milk. Add salt and pepper to taste. Pour into small oven-safe dish. Sprinkle with cheese. Bake for 10 minutes or until eggs are set. Enjoy OJ while you wait. Serve with toast and fruit butter.

CALORIES	471
FAT	18.2 GRAMS
CALCIUM	614 MG
FIBER	4.7 GRAMS

Midmorning Snack

½ cup Fiber One cereal with ½ cup skim milk

CALORIES	100
FAT	1 GRAM
CALCIUM	191 MG
FIBER	4.7 GRAMS

Lunch

CRAB-SALMON PATTY SANDWICH

1 tablespoon Dijonnaise
1 teaspoon white horseradish
1 whole-grain English muffin
1 crab-salmon patty
2 leaves **endive**
1 cup fresh or juice-packed **pineapple**

Combine Dijonnaise and horseradish. Set aside. Use fork to split English muffin. Toast until slightly brown. Top with crab-salmon patty, endive and horseradish-mustard sauce. Enjoy pineapple for dessert.

CALORIES	472
FAT	18.1 GRAMS
CALCIUM	424 MG
FIBER	6.2 GRAMS

Midafternoon Snack

1 oatmeal-raisin granola bar

CALORIES	130
FAT	2.3 GRAMS
CALCIUM	20 MG
FIBER	1.3 GRAMS

Dinner

SPINACH-CHEESE STRUDEL

1 teaspoon olive oil
½ teaspoon **garlic**, minced
1½ cups chopped fresh **spinach** (or ¾ cup frozen, thawed
   and drained)
Dash freshly ground pepper
Dash fresh **dill**
Dash nutmeg
½ cup part-skim ricotta or cottage cheese
Vegetable spray
2 sheets phyllo dough
1 wedge **watermelon**

Preheat oven to 350 degrees. Heat olive oil in pan and add garlic, spinach, pepper, dill and nutmeg. Cook until spinach is wilted. Remove from heat. Add ricotta or cottage cheese until well blended. Coat 8-inch pie pan or cake pan with vegetable spray. Remove 1 sheet phyllo dough from package and place in pan. Lightly coat sheet with vegetable spray. Place another sheet of phyllo on top and also coat with vegetable spray. Spoon in spinach mixture. Fold phyllo over top. Spray again and bake for 30 minutes, or until phyllo is brown. Serve with watermelon.

CALORIES	378
FAT	10 GRAMS
CALCIUM	280 MG
FIBER	8.6 GRAMS

TOTAL CALORIES FOR DAY 20	1,551
TOTAL FAT	49.6 GRAMS (29% OF TOTAL CALORIES)
TOTAL CALCIUM	1,529 MG
TOTAL FIBER	33.8 GRAMS

Day 21 SUNDAY

DENISEOLOGY
Don't take your health for granted—prevention is the best medicine.

THE GAME PLAN

- *Ahhhhh* . . . it's your rejuvenation day! You've worked hard all week—time to relax and unwind! Take the day off or enjoy some light movement—a stroll around town, some yoga moves or playing with your kids. You're doing an amazing job—keep up the good work.
- Today, choose Fidget-cizers that will help you relax, like waist twists, neck relaxers and shoulder stretches.

DAILY TIP

Use aromatherapy to create a spa atmosphere right in your own home. Scientists say that we can use certain smells to soothe or stimulate our spirits. Scents such as chamomile and lavender promote relaxation. Lemongrass, jasmine and rosemary invigorate. Sandalwood lifts spirits and promotes sensuality. Eucalyptus soothes achy muscles. You can buy scented oils at beauty-goods stores or drugstores. Try pouring them into your bath or dab them onto your pillow.

MEAL PLAN

Breakfast

BREAKFAST SANDWICH

    1 whole-grain English muffin
    2 slices **tomato**
    2 slices reduced-fat Alpine Lace Swiss cheese
    1 6-inch **banana**

Split English muffin in half and toast. Top each half with 1 slice tomato and 1 slice cheese. Broil until cheese melts. Serve with banana.

CALORIES	444
FAT	7.9 GRAMS
CALCIUM	542 MG
FIBER	8.5 GRAMS

Midmorning Snack

½ Florida **grapefruit**

CALORIES	40
FAT	0.1 GRAM
CALCIUM	14 MG
FIBER	6 GRAMS

Lunch

NACHOS

2 tablespoons water
½ small **onion,** finely chopped
¼ pound extra-lean turkey breast
¼ cup **picante sauce** or **salsa**
1 serving baked tortilla chips
1 tablespoon **salsa**
½ cup shredded **lettuce**
¼ cup shredded light cheddar cheese

Add water to nonstick pan. Add onion and turkey. Cook over medium heat until done, about 10 minutes. Add picante sauce or salsa. Spoon over tortilla chips and top with 1 tablespoon salsa, lettuce and cheese.

CALORIES	471
FAT	13.5 GRAMS
CALCIUM	585 MG
FIBER	2.8 GRAMS

Midafternoon Snack

1 box Cracker Jack

CALORIES	150
FAT	2.5 GRAMS
CALCIUM	0 MG
FIBER	1 GRAM

Dinner

FISH À L'ORANGE

1 4-ounce fillet orange roughy, cod, scrod or flounder
1 **orange**, sliced
¼ teaspoon grated orange peel
1 tablespoon fresh **parsley**, chopped
1 teaspoon olive oil
1 cup **broccoli**, steamed
Splash soy sauce
2 ears **corn**, fresh or frozen
2 tablespoons whipped butter

Preheat oven to 350 degrees. Place fish on large piece foil with orange slices, orange peel, parsley and olive oil. Close foil into a package and bake for 10 to 15 minutes. Steam broccoli and splash with soy sauce. Boil corn until warm and serve with whipped butter.

CALORIES	484
FAT	12 GRAMS
CALCIUM	106 MG
FIBER	12.13 GRAMS

TOTAL CALORIES FOR DAY 21	1,589
TOTAL FAT	36 GRAMS (20% OF TOTAL CALORIES)
TOTAL CALCIUM	1,247 MG
TOTAL FIBER	30.6 GRAMS

Week 3—Weekly Weigh-In

Hi! I'm just touching base with you—you're in the homestretch now! You should feel so proud of yourself.

Well, you've just finished 21 days . . . and scientists believe that it takes 21 days of repetition to form a habit. Yes—great habits! Thinking more positively, exercising regularly and even changing the way you eat.

Let's see how we're doing. Step on the scale first thing tomorrow morning (Monday—Day 22) before you eat or drink anything, preferably wearing only your "birthday suit."

Record Week 3 Weight

Day 22: _____ pounds

You are already a winner—you've taken a giant leap toward gaining control of your body and your life. Feel great? You should! Your self-confidence is soaring. You can do anything. So keep it up. Remember that this is just the beginning of a journey to a healthy new lifestyle.

By now, most of you should notice that you are stronger. You know what you're doing and you tackle your exercise routines with the strength and confidence of a lifelong athlete—something you couldn't even imagine during the first week. You are definitely moving toward a better body!

You may also be discovering that the greatest rewards of exercise are not even physical ones. You're less stressed. You fall asleep with ease. You have more energy. I bet you even notice a change in your personal life. Your kids say how much fun you are now. You wake up with a smile. Even professionally, you are more alert, productive, improved. Aren't the benefits of exercise wonderful?

Take on this last week with gusto! Make things happen. You have the power in you to change—not just your body but your whole attitude about life. I want you to finish out your last week a winner. It's up to you, because YOU ARE worth it! God gave us one body—take good care of both it and you. You can do it!

7 | Week Four

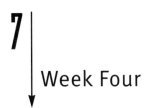

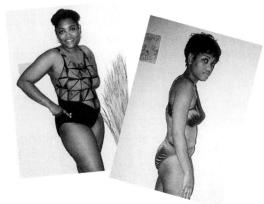

Monica lost
40 pounds and
three dress sizes.
*"After having five
children, I thought I
would never lose
weight. I had tried
different methods
and Denise's was
the only one that
worked. I am so
happy now!"*

WEEK AT A GLANCE

MONDAY: Cardio—Walk/jog intervals (30 minutes)
Mind-Body-Spirit Routine (5 minutes)

TUESDAY: Toning—Weight training (30 minutes)

WEDNESDAY: Cardio—Fat-Burning Blast with light weights
(30 minutes)
Mind-Body-Spirit Routine (5 minutes)

THURSDAY: Toning—Yoga and Pilates Method (30 minutes)

FRIDAY: Cardio—Triple cardio mix with muscle-toning circuit
(30 minutes)
Mind-Body-Spirit Routine (5 minutes)

SATURDAY: Play Day (60 minutes)

SUNDAY: Rejuvenation Day

You're almost there! You've made incredible progress—and you have just seven days to go. Part of you wants to ease up. But the finish line is in sight. I want you to race across it! This week, you'll be pushing even harder during your aerobic workouts. Ready to go for the gold? Let's move!

Thought of the Week: Count Your Blessings!

Did you ever get so annoyed with someone that you mentally added up all the little things that he or she ever did wrong? Then, because dwelling on the negatives got you all worked up, it took forever to forgive and resolve the situation?

We all tend to vent our hurts and disappointments when we feel let down by a friend, a sibling or even a coworker. But I've found a better way to resist the stress and negativity that can disrupt our relationships and waste valuable time.

When someone you are close to disappoints you, rather than counting all their mistakes and flaws, make a credit check of all his or her wonderful qualities. You'll find yourself gaining perspective as your list grows. Your tension subsides, and your mind is free to get back to happier, more productive thoughts.

Lists help you to prioritize your activities and remember what is most important to you. When my head is spinning from kids with sniffles to a tough TV taping to a nearly empty refrigerator, only lists can unscramble my day. And my most important list—the one that truly keeps me going—is my Count Our Blessings Every Day List!

I count my husband, Jeff, and daughters, Kelly and Katie, as well as my parents, my three sisters, my brother and all my friends. OK, I count my dog Madonna, too. I count our health. Our love. Our faith. Our professional achievements. And every beautiful morning I wake up with a smile and the energy to do it all.

I like to write my list down so I carry it with me at all times. Whenever I'm feeling hurt, disappointed or overwhelmed by work, I whip out the list and reflect on all I have to be thankful for. It serves as an instant sanity check!

Have you counted your blessings lately? When you do, include your smart commitment to losing weight and getting in shape. You have so many reasons to stay healthy and fit—among them your kids, spouse, parents, siblings and friends. And don't forget *you*. If you want to be successful in weight loss, you can't just do it for someone else—you have to do it for yourself, too. You deserve to feel strong and energetic so you can live life to the fullest!

Week 4 Shopping List

PRODUCE

8 mushrooms
2 plums
2 tomatoes
1 mango
1 red pepper
12-ounce bottle calcium-
  fortified orange juice
1 nectarine
4 new potatoes
1 zucchini

2 bananas
1 peach
½ pound sugar snap peas
1 small cucumber
2 pints mixed berries or
  1 pound frozen mixed
  berries
1 8-ounce can V-8 juice
10-ounce bag salad greens
1 cantaloupe

MEAT/PROTEIN

¼ pound extra-lean sirloin
1 4-ounce salmon fillet

1 package skinless chicken
  thighs
1 8-ounce filet mignon

MISCELLANEOUS

1 Boboli individual-size pizza
  crust

Day 22 MONDAY

THE GAME PLAN

• It's your fourth week—be thankful that you have a healthy body and think how absolutely wonderful you'll feel at the end of this week.

• Take on your 30-minute aerobic workout with confidence and purpose. You're much stronger and healthier than you were three weeks ago . . . so let me see it! Work harder as you walk, ride or run. If you decide to follow the usual walk/jog interval workout on pages 147 to 151, really push yourself. Make these 30 minutes work for you!

• Focus on toning your abs with today's Fidget-cizers. Do tummy tucks while you sit in the car or your office and crunches during TV commercials. (See pages 204 to 212.)

DAILY TIP

Music gets you moving . . . especially on days when you just don't feel like leaving the house. So make a tape of your favorite tunes. Some of my all-time favorites: *Change Would Do You Good* (Sheryl Crow), *One Week* (Barenaked Ladies), *Passionate Kisses* (Mary-Chapin Carpenter), *Cup of Life* (Ricky Martin), *Believe* (Cher), *I Will Survive* (Gloria Gaynor), *Respect* (Aretha Franklin).

MEAL PLAN

Breakfast

WAFFLES

> 2 frozen waffles
> ¼ cup whipped part-skim ricotta
> 1 teaspoon sugar
> Dash vanilla
> ½ cup fresh or frozen **mixed berries**

Warm waffles. Mix together ricotta, sugar and vanilla. Top waffles with ricotta mixture and berries.

CALORIES	284
FAT	7.5 GRAMS
CALCIUM	249 MG
FIBER	2.7 GRAMS

Midmorning Snack

10 dried **apricot** halves

CALORIES	83
FAT	0.2 GRAM
CALCIUM	16 MG
FIBER	3.1 GRAMS

Lunch

FRITATTA

1 teaspoon olive oil
2 tablespoons **onion**, finely chopped
1 cup total **mushrooms, zucchini,** and **baby spinach leaves,** chopped
5 green olives, chopped
2 eggs
1 tablespoon water
1 teaspoon Italian seasoning
Ground pepper, to taste
1 tablespoon grated Parmesan cheese
2 tablespoons **chunky pasta sauce**
1 whole-grain roll
1 tablespoon fruit butter
2 small **plums**

In a nonstick pan, heat olive oil. Add onion, vegetables and olives and sauté for 5 to 7 minutes. In a separate bowl, combine eggs, water, Italian seasoning and pepper; beat until thoroughly mixed. Pour eggs over vegetable mixture and cook on medium heat until set. Sprinkle Parmesan on top for flavor. Top with pasta sauce. Serve with roll and fruit butter. Enjoy plums for dessert.

CALORIES	469
FAT	23 GRAMS
CALCIUM	227 MG
FIBER	5.7 GRAMS

Midafternoon Snack

1 small, low-fat bran muffin

CALORIES	200
FAT	3 GRAMS
CALCIUM	66 MG
FIBER	3.9 GRAMS

Dinner

LEMON HERB-ROASTED CHICKEN THIGHS

2 small, skinless chicken thighs
1 **carrot**, chopped
2 3-inch-diameter **red potatoes**, halved
1 stalk **celery**, cut into 2-inch pieces
1 small **onion**, chopped
2 tablespoons low-fat lemon herb sauce
1 cup **mixed berries**
2 tablespoons low-fat whipped topping

Preheat oven to 350 degrees. In a baking pan, place chicken thighs, carrot, potatoes, celery and onion. Top with herb sauce. Cover with foil and bake for 30 minutes or until chicken is cooked through. For dessert, top berries with whipped topping and enjoy!

CALORIES	498
FAT	12 GRAMS
CALCIUM	39 MG
FIBER	15.2 GRAMS

TOTAL CALORIES FOR DAY 22	1,534
TOTAL FAT	45.7 GRAMS (27% OF TOTAL CALORIES)
TOTAL CALCIUM	597 MG
TOTAL FIBER	30.6 GRAMS

Day 23 TUESDAY

DENISEOLOGY
If you start doing with your body, your mind will follow.

THE GAME PLAN

• Remember, muscles burn more calories than fat! So turn to pages 154 to 166 for my weight-training workout. Today I want you to focus on working each muscle to the point of fatigue—so that at the end of each set, you absolutely can't lift the weight one more time. The harder you work, the more metabolism-boosting muscle you'll build.

• Fidget-cize! I know, it's become such a habit that you don't need to be reminded—but I will anyway!

DAILY TIP

Research shows that people who exercise regularly score higher on tests than those who don't. So march in place while watching *Jeopardy!*—you may just get that final answer right!

MEAL PLAN

Breakfast

BREAKFAST SANDWICH

2 slices multigrain bread, toasted
1 tablespoon natural chunky peanut butter
1 teaspoon honey
1 banana

Make sandwich with first three ingredients. Serve with banana.

CALORIES	292
FAT	9.6 GRAMS
CALCIUM	30 MG
FIBER	7 GRAMS

Midmorning Snack

CREAMSICLE

½ cup skim milk
4 ounces calcium-fortified **orange juice**
1 teaspoon honey
2 tablespoons wheat bran
3 ice cubes

Blend all ingredients until creamy.

CALORIES	107
FAT	0 GRAMS
CALCIUM	290 MG
FIBER	3.1 GRAMS

Lunch

TUNA PITA POCKET

1 3-ounce can water-packed tuna
2 tablespoons light mayonnaise
1 small whole-wheat pita
½ cup baby **carrots**
1 cup **vegetable soup**
1 **apple**

Combine tuna with mayonnaise. Fill pita and serve with carrots and soup. Follow up with the apple!

CALORIES	379
FAT	13 GRAMS
CALCIUM	58 MG
FIBER	10.3 GRAMS

Midafternoon Snack

1 serving baked tortilla chips (13 chips)
¼ cup fat-free **bean dip**
2 tablespoons **salsa**

CALORIES	170
FAT	1 GRAM
CALCIUM	40 MG
FIBER	4.4 GRAMS

Dinner

CHICKEN-VEGGIE PIZZA

½ boneless, skinless chicken breast
1 tablespoon light vinaigrette
1 cup total of **zucchini, mushrooms** and **red pepper**, cut
    into chunks
1 individual size Boboli pizza crust
2 tablespoons pesto sauce
½ cup canned **pineapple**

Preheat oven to 350 degrees. Grill chicken in vinaigrette. Cut into chunks when done. Grill vegetables for 5 minutes or roast them for 10 minutes. Spread pizza crust with pesto sauce and top with chicken and veggies. Bake for about 15 minutes, or until crust is crunchy. Have pineapple for dessert.

CALORIES	611
FAT	11.3 GRAMS
CALCIUM	22 MG
FIBER	3.6 GRAMS

TOTAL CALORIES FOR DAY 23	1,559
TOTAL FAT	35 GRAMS (20% OF TOTAL CALORIES)
TOTAL CALCIUM	709 MG
TOTAL FIBER	28.4 GRAMS

Day 24 WEDNESDAY

DENISEOLOGY
We all need to feel appreciated. So tell someone you love how much you treasure them today! A smile, a compliment, one kind sentence—those little things can make a person's day.

THE GAME PLAN
• Ready for another blast of fat-burning aerobics? Turn to pages 168 to 176 for your Fat-Burning Blast workout, or do any 30-minute workout of your choice. Focus on how you feel afterward. Your body feels strong and your mood is elevated. You're completely empowered. Whenever you're tempted to skip a workout, think about how great you feel when you're finished. It may be just the incentive you need!

• Did you Fidget-cize today? I'm counting—so make sure you move every hour!

DAILY TIP
Pretty your plate. Arrange your well-balanced meals so that you enjoy every fresh, flavorful forkful. Concentrate on enjoying quality instead of quantity.

MEAL PLAN

Breakfast

CEREAL

> 1 cup Multi-Grain Cheerios
> ¼ cup Fiber One
> ¾ cup skim milk
> 1 fresh **peach** or 1 cup frozen sliced **peaches**

Combine the above and greet the day with a smile!

CALORIES	237
FAT	1.5 GRAMS
CALCIUM	362 MG
FIBER	11.2 GRAMS

Midmorning Snack

1 oat-cinnamon granola bar

CALORIES	100
FAT	3 GRAMS
CALCIUM	0 MG
FIBER	1.5 GRAMS

Lunch

RICOTTA-BROCCOLI PASTA

¾ cup dry pasta (rotini, penne or radiatore)
½ cup part-skim ricotta
½ cup steamed **broccoli florets**
1 teaspoon olive oil
2 tablespoons grated Parmesan cheese
1 cup **mixed fresh or frozen berries**
Splash **cranberry juice**

Cook pasta until al dente. Add ricotta, broccoli and olive oil. Top with Parmesan cheese. Serve with berries splashed with cranberry juice.

CALORIES	546
FAT	10 GRAMS
CALCIUM	259 GRAMS
FIBER	11 GRAMS

Midafternoon Snack

2 frozen fruit bars

CALORIES	90
FAT	0 GRAMS
CALCIUM	0 MG
FIBER	0 GRAMS

Dinner

FILET AND VEGETABLES

1 4-ounce filet mignon
1 teaspoon **garlic,** minced
Splash Worcestershire sauce
Dash Italian seasoning
4 1-inch-diameter **new potatoes,** peeled
1 teaspoon olive oil
½ teaspoon rosemary leaves
1 cup **mixed vegetables**
½ cup **natural applesauce**

Preheat oven to 500 degrees. Season filet with garlic, Worcestershire sauce and Italian seasoning. Broil until pink in the middle, about 5 minutes per side. In a nonstick skillet, sauté potatoes in olive oil and rosemary for about 5 minutes, until lightly browned. Cover and cook over low heat for about 10 minutes or until tender (to prevent potatoes from sticking or burning, you may want to add enough chicken broth or water to cover the bottom of the pan). Steam vegetables. Serve applesauce on the side or for dessert.

CALORIES	511
FAT	20 GRAMS
CALCIUM	78 MG
FIBER	4.3 GRAMS

TOTAL CALORIES FOR DAY 24	1,484
TOTAL FAT	34.5 GRAMS (21% OF TOTAL CALORIES)
TOTAL CALCIUM	699 MG
TOTAL FIBER	28 GRAMS

Day 25 THURSDAY

DENISEOLOGY
Laugh hard—it's the best medicine and it tightens the tummy!

THE GAME PLAN

- As you've noticed by now, I hope, muscles work miracles on your metabolism! Turn to pages 179 to 193 for your yoga- and Pilates-based toning workout.
- Are you keeping up with your Fidget-cizing? Pick your least favorite move from pages 204 to 212 and do it now. No complaining!

DAILY TIP

Go in search of a little humor today—it's terrific for both the body and the spirit. When I need to do a good belly laugh, I turn on *I Love Lucy* reruns and crack up. Watching Lucy and Ethel in the chocolate factory helps me forget my worries and works my abs at the same time.

MEAL PLAN

Breakfast

EGG SANDWICH

>   1 egg
>   Vegetable spray
>   1 whole-grain English muffin, toasted
>   1 slice Muenster or Gouda cheese
>   1 **orange**

Fry egg in nonstick skillet coated with vegetable spray. Place on English muffin and top with cheese. Cut orange into wedges and enjoy!

CALORIES	304
FAT	15 GRAMS
CALCIUM	269 MG
FIBER	7.5 GRAMS

Midmorning Snack

1 2-inch **watermelon wedge**

CALORIES   51
FAT   0 GRAMS
CALCIUM   13 MG
FIBER   0.8 GRAMS

Lunch

STIR-FRY VEGGIE TORTILLAS

1 teaspoon olive oil
½ teaspoon grated ginger
½ teaspoon **garlic**, minced
1 small green **onion**, chopped
1 cup frozen **Oriental vegetables**
Soy sauce, to taste
2 flour tortillas
Plum sauce
1 **nectarine**

Heat olive oil in skillet. Add ginger, garlic and onion. Add Oriental veggies and sauté until crisp-tender. Add soy sauce to taste. Spread flour tortillas with plum sauce. Spoon veggies into tortillas. Follow it up with a nectarine.

CALORIES   482.5
FAT   10.4 GRAMS
CALCIUM   145 MG
FIBER   8.8 GRAMS

Midafternoon Snack

8 ounces **V-8 juice**
½ multigrain bagel topped with 1 tablespoon light cream cheese

CALORIES   169
FAT   2.9 GRAMS
CALCIUM   44 MG
FIBER   2.6 GRAMS

Dinner

LASAGNA ROLLS

¼ pound extra-lean ground beef or ground turkey breast
Salt and pepper to taste
1 cup total **spinach, mushrooms, zucchini** and **peppers,**
    chopped
2 lasagna noodles
½ cup low-fat cottage cheese
½ cup **chunky pasta sauce**
2 cups **mixed greens**
2 tablespoons light raspberry vinaigrette

Brown meat and season with salt and pepper as desired. Add chopped veggies. Set aside. Boil lasagna noodles until al dente. Mix meat mixture with cottage cheese. Lay flat one lasagna noodle; spread length of noodle with half of the meat mixture and roll up. Repeat with second noodle and remainder of meat mixture. Place in baking pan. Top rolls with pasta sauce. Toss greens with vinaigrette and serve.

CALORIES	556
FAT	19.9 GRAMS
CALCIUM	125 MG
FIBER	5.4 GRAMS

TOTAL CALORIES FOR DAY 25	1,562.5
TOTAL FAT	48.2 GRAMS (28% OF TOTAL CALORIES)
TOTAL CALCIUM	596 MG
TOTAL FIBER	25.1 GRAMS

Day 26 FRIDAY

THE GAME PLAN

• Time to really blast the fat! Turn to pages 195 to 202 for your Circuit Training workout, or do 30 minutes of the aerobic activity of your choice. While you're moving, think about your workouts for next week. Our 28 days may be almost over, but if you want to keep those 10 pounds off, you have to keep going. Your health depends on it!

• TGIF = Thank Goodness I Fidget-cize! And while you're giving thanks, don't forget to fidget!

DAILY TIP

Be flexible! If bad weather interferes with your usual four-mile power walk or a business trip means no equipment for your weight-training workout, don't just say "Forget it." Always have a backup plan, such as doing an exercise video or push-ups and triceps dips in your hotel room. Trying a new workout will be great for your body and your psyche—and you'll feel inspired to keep your workout streak going!

MEAL PLAN

Breakfast

> 1 tablespoon natural chunky peanut butter
> 1 tablespoon honey
> 1 slice multigrain bread, toasted
> ½ **Florida grapefruit**

Top toast with peanut butter and honey. Serve grapefruit on the side.

CALORIES	266
FAT	9.1 GRAMS
CALCIUM	42 MG
FIBER	8 GRAMS

Midmorning Snack

1 cup Multi-Grain Cheerios with 5 **dried apricots** and 1
tablespoon slivered almonds

CALORIES	237
FAT	8.7 GRAMS
CALCIUM	83 MG
FIBER	5.8 GRAMS

Lunch

VEGGIE BURGER

1 soy-based veggie burger
1 multigrain roll
2 tablespoons **salsa**
½ cup **endive** or **romaine lettuce**
2 tablespoons reduced-fat cheddar cheese, shredded
½ **cantaloupe**

Grill, broil or microwave veggie burger. Place on roll and top
with salsa, endive or lettuce, and cheese. Broil until cheese
melts. Serve cantaloupe for dessert.

CALORIES	399
FAT	12.1 GRAMS
CALCIUM	250 MG
FIBER	9.3 GRAMS

Midafternoon Snack

4 ounces fruit-flavored low-fat yogurt
1 cup frozen or fresh **blackberries** or **raspberries**

CALORIES	187
FAT	1.3 GRAMS
CALCIUM	180 MG
FIBER	7.6 GRAMS

Dinner

SALMON FILLET

> 1 4-ounce salmon fillet or salmon steak
> Dash Old Bay seasoning
> 1 cup prepared risotto
> 1 cup **sugar snap peas**

Sprinkle salmon with Old Bay seasoning. Broil or grill until done. Prepare risotto according to package. Steam sugar snap peas. A wonderful meal!

CALORIES	496
FAT	15.3 GRAMS
CALCIUM	69 MG
FIBER	2 GRAMS

TOTAL CALORIES FOR DAY 26	1,585
TOTAL FAT	46.5 GRAMS (26% OF TOTAL CALORIES)
TOTAL CALCIUM	624 MG
TOTAL FIBER	32.7 GRAMS

Day 27 SATURDAY

THE GAME PLAN

- I want you to really enjoy your Free Day. So make it a day filled with activities that you love! Hike to a waterfall, then spend five minutes soaking in the lush scenery and the sound of falling water. Organize a softball game. Plan a group hike or go skiing with friends. Taking time to smell the roses doesn't mean you should ignore your need to move. As you now know, you *can* do both.
- While you're deciding how to spend your day, don't forget to Fidget-cize. And while you smell the roses, do a few squats!

DAILY TIP

Your tootsies need attention, too! Try this wonderful treat for aching feet: Sit on the edge of a bed or a chair and place a tennis or golf ball on the floor. Center your foot on top of the ball and roll it from side to side, then forward and backward. After massaging for a minute, switch feet and repeat.

MEAL PLAN

Breakfast

    8 ounces yogurt
    1 low-fat granola bar
    1 6-inch **banana**

CALORIES	460
FAT	4.9 GRAMS
CALCIUM	341 MG
FIBER	4 GRAMS

Midmorning Snack

1 cup herbal tea with ¼ cup **cranberry juice** added

CALORIES	20
FAT	0 GRAMS
CALCIUM	0 GRAMS
FIBER	0 GRAMS

Lunch

FAJITA PITA

1 teaspoon olive oil
1 4-ounce turkey breast fillet or chicken breast
½ cup sliced **yellow, red,** or **orange peppers**
½ cup sliced **onion**
2 tablespoons fajita sauce
1 whole-wheat pita
2 tablespoons **picante sauce**
1 **apple**

In nonstick skillet, heat olive oil, then add meat, peppers, onion and fajita sauce. Sauté until meat is cooked. Serve in pita with picante sauce. Crunch an apple for dessert!

CALORIES	417
FAT	9.7 GRAMS
CALCIUM	19 MG
FIBER	8.3 GRAMS

Midafternoon Snack

1 **orange**

CALORIES	60
FAT	1 GRAM
CALCIUM	52 MG
FIBER	3.1 GRAMS

Dinner

TORTELLINI AND VEGETABLES

⅓ package light cheese tortellini
1 cup **green beans**
1 tablespoon slivered almonds
1 teaspoon whipped butter
¾ cup **chunky pasta sauce**
1 tablespoon grated Parmesan cheese
½ **mango,** cut into strips

Prepare tortellini according to package. Steam green beans. Sauté almonds in butter and add to beans. Top tortellini with pasta sauce and cheese. Enjoy the mango for dessert!

CALORIES	609.5
FAT	18.9 GRAMS
CALCIUM	327 MG
FIBER	10.1 GRAMS

TOTAL CALORIES FOR DAY 27	1,566.5
TOTAL FAT	34.5 GRAMS (20% OF TOTAL CALORIES)
TOTAL CALCIUM	739 MG
TOTAL FIBER	25.5 GRAMS

Day 28 SUNDAY

> ## DENISEOLOGY
> *Feeling good about yourself involves more than a fit body. Commit yourself to constant self-improvement by challenging your mind as well as your body . . . and savor that feeling of self-accomplishment!*

THE GAME PLAN

• WOW! What more can I say? You did it! No matter how much weight you lost, the last 28 days have been a great success! You've created new healthy habits that I want you to keep for a lifetime. And now that you're programmed to move and eat right, your metabolism should stay supercharged—and the weight should stay off. In Chapter 15, I'll address some of the obstacles that you may face down the road. Maintaining a healthy weight doesn't have to be hard—and it's 100 percent doable. Remember: This isn't a diet, it's a *lifestyle*. So get out there and live!

• Make your new habits stick—Fidget-cize every day as often as you can!

DAILY TIP

Give yourself a treat that you don't eat. You've worked hard and deserve a reward—earrings, fresh flowers, your favorite magazine, or better still, some new workout gear!

MEAL PLAN

Breakfast

PARISIAN CAFÉ BREAKFAST

1 8-ounce café latte made with skim milk or 8 ounces skim milk
1 small, low-fat bran muffin or ½ large low-fat bran muffin

CALORIES	280
FAT	4 GRAMS
CALCIUM	307 MG
FIBER	5 GRAMS

Midmorning Snack

¼ cup Fiber One with 2 tablespoons **raisins**

CALORIES	89
FAT	0.5 GRAM
CALCIUM	20 MG
FIBER	7.9 GRAMS

Lunch

BLACK BEAN SOUP AND TOMATO SALAD

1 medium **tomato,** cubed
1 tablespoon light vinaigrette
1 8-ounce can **black bean soup**
⅓ cup cooked brown rice
1 tablespoon **green onions,** chopped
1 tablespoon light sour cream
½ Florida **grapefruit**

Toss tomato with light vinaigrette. Let salad sit so flavor sets. Heat soup. Add rice and top with onions and sour cream. Have grapefruit for dessert.

CALORIES	445
FAT	8 GRAMS
CALCIUM	52 MG
FIBER	12.3 GRAMS

Midafternoon Snack

1 Denise Austin's Tasty Meal-to-Go bar, any flavor

CALORIES	220
FAT	5 GRAMS
CALCIUM	350 MG
FIBER	2 GRAMS

Dinner

GRILLED STEAK SALAD

1 4-ounce filet mignon, strip or sirloin steak
2 cups **romaine lettuce**
$1/2$ **cucumber**, chopped
$1/2$ **sweet pepper**, sliced, or $1/4$ cup **roasted red pepper**
2 tablespoons light vinaigrette
1 4-inch baguette
$1/2$ teaspoon olive oil
Sprinkle Italian seasoning
Dash garlic powder or $1/2$ **garlic** clove, minced
Sprinkle Parmesan cheese

Grill or broil beef. Slice into finger-size strips. Toss lettuce, cucumber, peppers and vinaigrette. Top with beef. Split baguette in half. Brush each side with olive oil. Sprinkle with Italian seasoning, garlic and cheese. Broil until cheese melts. A great way to end our 28 days!

CALORIES	514
FAT	19.7 GRAMS
CALCIUM	116 MG
FIBER	4 GRAMS

TOTAL CALORIES FOR DAY 28	1,548
TOTAL FAT	37 GRAMS (22% OF TOTAL CALORIES)
TOTAL CALCIUM	845 MG
TOTAL FIBER	31 GRAMS

Week 4—Weekly Weigh-In

Congratulations! Give yourself a standing ovation! You did it. No matter how much weight you lost, you're a winner. The fact that you made the decision to improve yourself and get healthy makes you one. Now you're thriving—not simply surviving.

Tomorrow morning you will be stepping on that scale and remeasuring yourself to see your results. Remember not to eat or drink anything before weighing in, and hit the scale wearing only your "birthday suit."

Record Week 4 Weight

Day 29: _____ pounds

Now get out your measuring tape and remeasure yourself in those five areas of the body as you did on Day 1.

Measurements

  1. Upper arm: Right: _____ inches

                                     Left: _____ inches

  2. Chest (across your bustline):   _____ inches

  3. Waistline: _____ inches

  4. Hips (around the widest point):   _____ inches

  5. Thighs (around the widest point):   _____ inches

So how did you do? Did you reach your goal? Did you lose inches? I hope you feel mentally and physically strong as well as lighter in pounds and inches. The best part of all is the belief in yourself that you know you can do it! I want you to feel proud of your successes and accomplishments.

If you haven't lost those last 10 pounds, please don't feel like you failed. You didn't. Just keep going for it! With my plan, you've been given all the tools that you need to reach your true potential. You can do it!!!

For the past four weeks, you've worked hard to transform negative habits into positive new ones. The key to maintaining all those healthy habits is to keep living them every day. Staying on track and remaining in control of your decision to eat right, exercise regularly and think positively should be your goal for life. The whole point of my program was to introduce you to some simple strategies that can be incorporated into the lifestyle of every normal, average person—like me and like you.

Post these basic tips in an obvious place as quick reminders of your new fit and healthy lifestyle:

1. **Eat in moderation.** I eat well 80 percent of the time and enjoy treats 20 percent of the time.
2. **Try not to eat late at night.** I try to allow three hours to help metabolize my dinner before bed.
3. **Drink plenty of water.** Water is critical to help metabolize fat.
4. **Be a smart shopper.** I try to shop the perimeter of the grocery store first, because that is where all the fresh produce, meats, fish and low-fat dairy products are located. Plus I read labels for fat, sodium and fiber content. Nothing enters my basket that I haven't read about first.
5. **Don't be afraid to ask questions when dining out.** I believe in ordering exactly what you want. So ask how foods are cooked—don't be embarrassed to take control!
6. **Keep moving!** I work out almost every day for 30 minutes. Schedule those activities into your calendar. And don't forget to Fidget-cize!
7. **Be positive!** Be proud! You are a unique, beautiful person—the one and only you! Be confident, heathier and happier. You are worth it!

Part 3

The Workouts

8

Monday: Walk/Jog Intervals

In recent years, interval training has been a hot trend in the fitness world. Everyone from Olympic athletes to Hollywood's A-list is using interval training to improve their performance and shed body fat—fast! With interval training, you alternate bursts of high-intensity exercise ("work") with low-intensity exercise ("recovery"). The goal is to really push yourself during the "work" portion of each interval and then ease up briefly to let your body "recover" and bring your heart rate back down to prepare for the next round of high-intensity activity.

This type of high/low intensity training actually burns fat much more effectively than a continuous moderate-intensity workout. Why? Because rather than exercising at a comfortable level, you push your heart rate almost to its maximum—the key to burning more calories. By allowing yourself to catch your breath and recover, you're able to sustain an elevated pace for longer—and your metabolism remains supercharged both during and after your workout. Don't worry about the "calories burned" figure on your treadmill or stationary bike, which may seem lower than what you'd hoped for. Since your metabolism remains revved for up to *four hours* after interval training, you're burning many more calories than you realize!

Interval training is such a time-efficient, fat-busting workout that I do it at least once a week—and you will, too, over the next 28 days. To ensure that you continue to make progress, the walk/jog workout outlined on the following pages gets more and more intense throughout the program. In other words, you'll spend more time working and less time recovering with each workout. My program is all about becoming stronger, getting in better shape and moving forward in a positive way.

Intervals translate to most forms of exercise—you can do them whether you're riding a bike (think spinning), using a stair climber or rowing machine, or swimming laps. Feel free to take the principles of today's walk/jog interval workout and apply them to your favorite aerobic activity! These days, many cardio machines, including treadmills, stair climbers and stationary bikes, have built-in interval programs to make it easy for you. Or use the following guidelines to create your own workout and alter your intensity:

Speed up and speed down
Add and lower resistance
Change your terrain (i.e., go up and down hills)

The best way to monitor your intensity is to use a heart-rate monitor. As your intensity goes up, so does your heart rate. You also can use this Rate of Perceived Exertion Scale: On a scale of 1 to 10 (1 being the equivalent of lying on the couch and 10 being sprinting as fast as you can), aim for a 4 or 5 during the low-intensity portion of each interval and a 7 or 8 during the high-intensity portion.

If you're a beginner (you've never exercised or have been largely inactive for three months or more) or you have bad knees, simply walk as fast as you can during the work portion of your intervals. Your ultimate goal, however, is to jog or run. The higher you get your heart rate up, the more efficient and fat-busting your workout will be. If you can't run yet, don't fret—you can work up to it bit by bit. Just think of how accomplished and energized you'll feel when you are finally able to run for 30 minutes straight.

Since you'll be timing your intervals, make sure you have a watch or a clock handy. At the end of each workout, spend a few minutes doing the lower-body stretches on pages 149 to 150—they're critical to preventing soreness and injury. Follow each weekly interval workout with the two tummy-tightening exercises pictured on pages 150 to 151.

Reminder: If you already have a favorite aerobic workout, feel free to stick with it. This walk/jog interval workout is just another option for people who want to try something new and different. For a list of other fabulous fat-burning cardio workouts, see pages 168 to 174.

Week 1

For today's workout, you'll do six intervals total, alternating 3 minutes of low-intensity walking with 1 minute of high-intensity jogging or power walking. At the end, walk for 6 minutes to let your body cool down. Then do your lower-body stretches followed by ab work.

Day at a Glance

30-MINUTE INTERVAL WORKOUT
> **Interval ratio:** 3:1 (3 minutes of walking followed by 1 minute of jogging)
> **Number of intervals:** 6
> **Cool-down:** 6 minutes of walking

STRETCHES
> Quads, calves and hips/hamstrings

AB FIRMERS
> Total Tummy Tightener, Waist Trimmer

Week 2

For today's workout, you'll do eight intervals total, alternating 2 minutes of low-intensity walking with 1 minute of high-intensity jogging or fast walking. At the end, walk for 6 minutes to let your body cool down. Then, do your lower-body stretches followed by ab work.

Day at a glance

30-MINUTE INTERVAL WORKOUT
> **Interval ratio:** 2:1 (2 minutes of walking followed by 1 minute of jogging)
> **Number of intervals:** 8
> **Cool-down:** 6 minutes of walking

STRETCHES
> Quads, calves and hips/hamstrings

AB FIRMERS
> Total Tummy Tightener, Waist Trimmer

Week 3

For today's workout, you'll do five intervals total, alternating 3 minutes of low- intensity walking with 2 minutes of high-intensity jogging or fast walking. At the end, walk for 5 minutes to let your body cool down. Then do your lower-body stretches followed by ab work.

Day at a Glance

30-MINUTE INTERVAL WORKOUT
Interval ratio: 3:2 (3 minutes of walking followed by 2 minutes of jogging)
Number of intervals: 5
Cool-down: 5 minutes of walking

STRETCHES
Quads, calves and hips/hamstrings

AB FIRMERS
Total Tummy Tightener, Waist Trimmer

Week 4

For today's workout, you'll do six intervals total, alternating 2 minutes of low-intensity walking with 2 minutes of high-intensity jogging or fast walking. At the end, walk for 6 minutes to let your body cool down. Then do your lower-body stretches followed by ab work.

Day at a Glance

30-MINUTE INTERVAL WORKOUT
Interval ratio: 2:2 (2 minutes of walking followed by 2 minutes of jogging)
Number of intervals: 6
Cool-down: 6 minutes of walking

STRETCHES
Quads, calves and hips/hamstrings

AB FIRMERS
Total Tummy Tightener, Waist Trimmer

Walking Stretches

Quad Stretch

Stand with one hand holding a chair, a wall or a tree for balance. Lift your right foot behind you, then reach back and grab it with your right hand. Gently pull your heel toward your buttocks. Feel the stretch in the front of your thigh. Hold for 15 to 30 seconds, then switch legs and repeat.

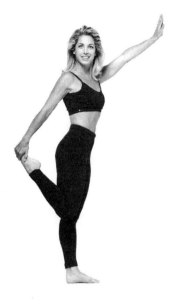

Calf Stretch

Stand facing a wall or a tree with one foot in front of the other (front foot is about 1 foot from the wall and back foot is about 3 feet from the wall). Keeping heels on the floor, place your hands on the wall in front of you and lean forward, bending your front knee. Feel the stretch in the back of the leg that is extended behind you. Hold for 15 to 30 seconds. Switch legs and repeat.

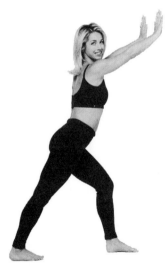

Hips/Hamstring Stretch

Lie on your back with your buttocks up against a wall. Extend one leg up so foot rests against the wall (leg forms a 90-degree angle from your torso); the other leg should be bent so that your outside ankle is resting on your thigh. Now slowly bend the knee of the leg against the wall. Hold for 15 to 30 seconds, then switch legs and repeat.

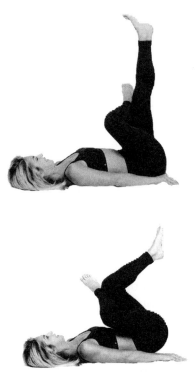

Ab Firmers

Total Tummy Tightener

Lie on your back with knees
bent and lifted so they're above
your hips. Place hands behind
ears to lightly support neck.
Exhale as you curl your upper
body toward your knees so your
shoulders lift off the floor
slightly; pull your belly button
in toward your spine. Inhale as
you release and lower your
shoulders to the floor. Do two
sets of 15 to 20 reps.

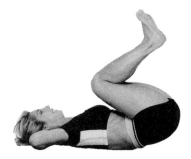

Waist Trimmer

Lying on your back, bend your
knees and elevate your feet
(advanced: extend your legs as
shown). Lift your left shoulder
off the floor and reach both
hands toward the outside of
your right knee. "Pulse" for
15 to 20 reps. Inhale as you
return to starting position, then
exhale as you reach both hands
toward the outside of your left
knee. "Pulse" for another 15 to
20 reps. Do a total of two sets
on each side.

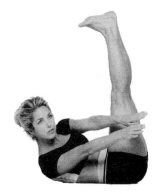

9

Tuesday: Weight Training

I started weight training in my early 20s, and I'm convinced that it's the reason I've been able to defy the aging process. Even though I recently turned 43, I feel like I'm 20! Lucky for all of you, accumulating research shows it's never too late to start working with weights and experiencing the many benefits of this type of workout.

Why look your age when you don't have to? Lifting weights is one of the best ways to fight gravity!

This 30-minute toning routine targets every area of your body, including your butt, thighs, shoulders, arms and abs. It features good, old-fashioned weight training moves, such as squat lunges and push-ups. If you've already spent some time in a weight room, you may recognize these exercises—they're some of the best, and they'll do wonders for your shape.

Women will need a set of 3-, 5- and 8-pound weights; men will need 8-, 10-, 12- or 15-pound weights. If you don't already own dumbbells, I highly recommend investing in a set. You can buy them at most major sporting-goods stores, and they are fairly inexpensive. However, if your budget prevents you from making this purchase, substitute household items such as soup cans or water bottles.

Many women hesitate to use weights because they're afraid that they'll bulk up—and go up a dress size instead of down. As I mentioned earlier, most of us simply don't have enough testosterone to become as big as bodybuilders. On the contrary, since working out with weights can help you get firm and lose flab, you'll probably lose body mass! Fat takes up five times as much space as muscle.

For each move, you'll want to use enough weight to challenge your muscles but not so much that you tire out quickly and your form gets sloppy. Each exercise should be smooth and controlled; the aim is to move the weight through a full range of motion. It's important not to hold your breath. Instead, you want to exhale on exertion and inhale on release. At the end of a set, your target muscles should feel fatigued and challenged (but not sore), which means that they're working and developing. If not, switch to a heavier weight. Your goal for the next four weeks is to *build* muscle, so you want to add a little weight as you get stronger.

I love to work out with my husband Jeff (yes, he's the handsome guy in these photos!), but you can do all of these exercises with or without a partner. For most of these moves, I'm using 5- to 8-pound weights and Jeff is using 10-pound weights; on page 155 I've provided suggested weight ranges depending on your fitness level. If you prefer following along with a video, pick up a copy of *Totally Firm: A Workout with Weights*—it's very similar to the workout on the next few pages.

Determine your level of experience and then refer to the chart (on page 155) to find the appropriate weight range. You're a beginner if you've never weight trained before or haven't done so in three or more months. You're intermediate if you've been weight training for only three months or so, and advanced if you've been weight training for a while.

Before starting, be sure to do three minutes of light cardio activity—marching in place, walking or jumping rope—to warm up your muscles and get your blood pumping. A proper warm-up will help you get more out of this workout and prevent injuries!

Ready to start developing those metabolism-boosting muscles? Remember: The waif look is out—toned is in! Plus, strong muscles are your best defense against aging. If your muscles are toned and taut, *nothing* can droop or sag. These age-defying exercises can help shrink middle-age spread, firm up sagging arms, and lift and tone your chest and buns!

Remember: This weight-loss plan is meant to work *with* you, not against you. Even though this is your weight-training day, if you're really craving a cardio workout, go for it! After 20 to 30 minutes of aerobics, take 10 minutes to do the toning exercises I have planned for today. You can do them immediately after your cardio or wait until later in the day. Or simply save today's workout for another day this week.

Lower Body

For each of these lower-body moves, do one set of 15 to 20 repetitions. After you've completed all six moves (which should take about five minutes), repeat the entire circuit again.

Squats

Holding a weight in each hand, stand with your feet a little wider than your hips, arms by your sides with elbows slightly bent. Keeping your back straight and abs tight, bend your knees and sit back into a squat, keeping your body weight over your heels. Your thighs should be as close to parallel to the floor as possible. Squeeze your buttocks as you straighten your legs to return to starting position, then repeat. If you have a history of knee problems, begin with a partial squat, with knees bent at about 45-degree angles. As you progress, never go lower than a 90-degree angle. *Benefits: Strengthens buttocks and thighs.*

Lift your buns as well as your spirits!

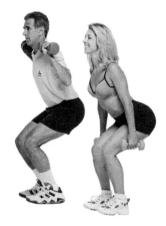

As you feel stronger, do these squats with your elbows bent and your hands at shoulder level—like Jeff.

HOW MUCH WEIGHT SHOULD YOU USE?
Beginner
WOMEN: Try the exercises without weights for the first week, then switch to 1- to 3-pound weights.
MEN: 8- to 10-pound weights
Intermediate
WOMEN: 3- to 5-pound weights
MEN: 10- to 12-pound weights
Advanced
WOMEN: 5- to 8-pound weights
MEN: 12-pound weights and up

Lunges

Holding a weight in each hand, stand with your feet about shoulder-width apart, arms by your sides. Take a big step forward with your right foot [A]. Slowly bend your right knee to a 90-degree angle, so your knee is directly above your ankle. Your weight should be balanced between the toes of your left foot and your right heel; don't let your back knee rest on the floor [B]. Straighten your right leg, pushing from your heel, to return to starting position. Do 15 to 20 reps. Switch sides and repeat with the opposite leg. *Benefits: Strengthens thighs and buttocks.*

Again, as you feel stronger, do these squats with your elbows bent and your hands at shoulder level—as Jeff is doing.

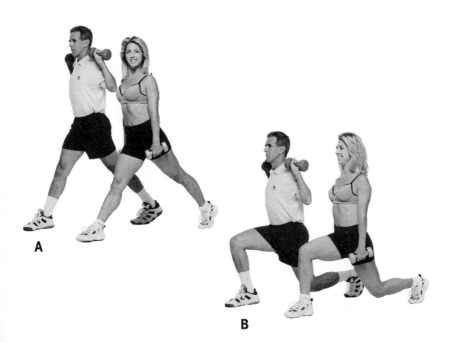

A

B

Dead Lifts

Holding a weight in each hand, stand with your feet shoulder-width apart, knees slightly bent [A]. Keeping your back flat and your knees slightly bent, bend forward at your hips to lower the weights toward the floor, your hands directly under your shoulders [B]. Don't expect the weights to reach the floor until your flexibility and strength improve. Slowly lift from your hips to return to an upright position, then repeat. *Benefits: Strengthens and lengthens your legs, especially your hamstrings (backs of thighs).*

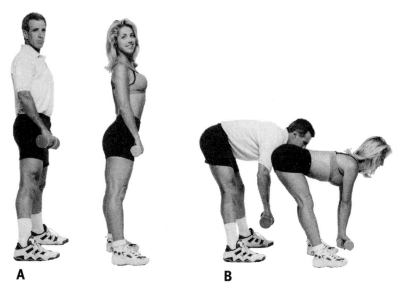

A   **B**

Outer-Thigh Lifts

Lie on the floor on your left side, left elbow planted on the floor directly beneath your shoulder, left knee bent, right hand on the floor in front of you for balance. Keeping your foot flexed, slowly raise your right leg, keeping it straight, about two feet off the floor; this is a very small movement, so be careful not to raise your leg too high [A]. Focus on the tension in your outer

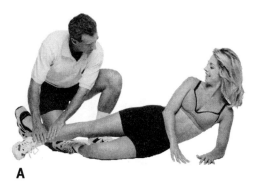

A

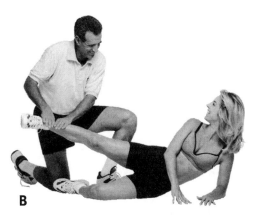

B

thigh. Complete all reps with your right leg, then switch sides and repeat with your left leg. As you grow accustomed to this exercise, add resistance: If you're working out with a partner, ask him or her to press on the leg you're raising [B]; if you're working out alone, use your free hand (hold a light dumbbell, if you're ready) to press down on your leg. *Benefits: Strengthens outer hips and thighs.*

Inner-Thigh Lifts

Lie on the floor on your left side, your left elbow planted on the floor directly beneath your shoulder, your right hand on the floor in front of you for balance. Bend your right leg and place your foot on the floor behind your left leg. Slowly raise your left leg off the floor to a comfortable height, keeping your leg as straight as possible. Pause at the top of the movement, then lower your leg back to the floor. Your left foot should remain flexed and parallel to the floor throughout the movement. Do all reps, then switch sides and repeat with the opposite leg. To add resistance, ask your partner or use your right hand (you can hold a light dumbbell or an ankle weight, if you're ready) to press down on the leg you're raising. *Benefits: Strengthens and tones inner thighs.*

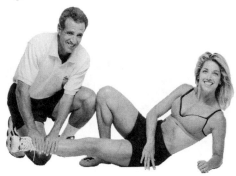

Glute Lifts

Kneel on the floor on all fours, hands directly beneath your shoulders, knees beneath your hips. Keeping your back flat, abs tight and hips square to the floor, raise your right leg, keeping it bent at a 90-degree angle, until your thigh is parallel to the floor. Slowly lower your knee back down to the floor, then up again, pressing your foot toward the ceiling and squeezing your buttocks. Continue alternating sides for all reps. To add resistance, ask your partner to press down on your foot as you lift and up on the top of your foot as you lower or use an ankle weight. *Benefits: Strengthens buttocks.*

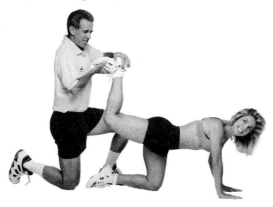

Upper Body

Do one set of 15 to 20 repetitions for each upper-body move. After you complete all six moves (which should take about five minutes), repeat the entire circuit again.

Push-ups

Kneel with your hands out in front of you on the floor. Supporting yourself on your hands, straighten your legs and rest your body weight on your toes; straighten your back, with your abs

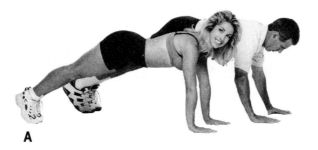

A

tight and your head in a natural position [A]. Slowly bend your elbows and lower your chest to the floor [B]. Straighten your elbows to return to starting position. Repeat. *Benefits: Strengthens chest, shoulders, triceps and abdominals.*

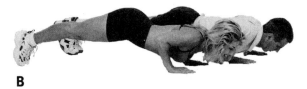

B

Modification: If straight-leg push-ups are too challenging, do bent-knee push-ups instead: Kneeling on the floor with your ankles crossed, repeat the same motion as above. As you develop upper-body strength, try switching to the straight-leg push-ups pictured above.

Chest Flies

You can do this exercise using a weight bench or on the floor. Sit on an incline bench or lie on your back on a flat weight bench with your feet flat on the floor; if you're on the floor, bend your knees and place your feet flat on the floor and place a pillow under your upper back. Holding a weight in each hand, extend your arms straight up, so your hands are directly above your shoulders [A]. Keeping arms slightly bent, slowly lower your arms to your sides; don't let the weights drop below your shoulders [B]. Squeeze your chest as you slowly raise the weights back to the starting position, and repeat. *Benefits: Strengthens chest, fronts of arms (biceps).*

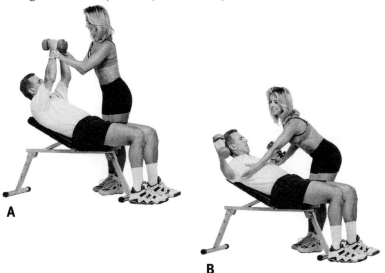

A

B

Bent-Over Rows

Holding a weight in each hand, stand with your feet shoulder-width apart, knees slightly bent. Keep your abs tight and back flat as you bend slightly forward at the hips; your arms should be at your sides and slightly in front of your torso. Squeeze your shoulder blades together as you lift your elbows so your upper arms are almost parallel to the floor, keeping elbows in 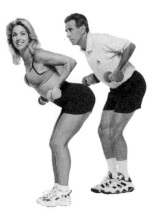 close to your body. Slowly return to starting position, and repeat. *Benefits: Strengthens upper back, backs of arms (triceps).*

Lat Pull-Downs

Sit on a bench or armless chair with your feet flat on the floor. Keep your back straight and your abs tight. Holding a weight in each hand, raise your arms over your head, palms facing forward [**A**]. Squeeze your shoulder blades down and together as you slowly bend your elbows, lowering the weights to shoulder level [**B**]. Squeeze shoulder blades together again as you slowly lift weights back up to starting position. *Benefits: Strengthens upper back (latissimus dorsi)—no more bra bulge!*

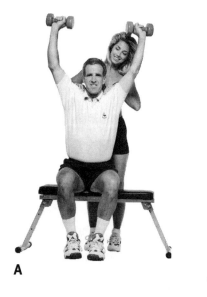

A

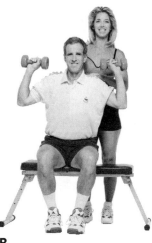

B

Lateral Raises

Holding a 5-pound dumbbell in each hand, stand with your feet shoulder-width apart, abs tight, back straight and knees slightly bent. Weights should be in front of you, palms facing toward you [A]. Bend your elbows slightly as you raise the weights out to your sides to shoulder height, palms facing down [B]. Slowly return to starting position, and repeat. *Benefits: Strengthens shoulders.*

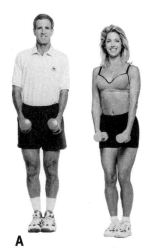

A

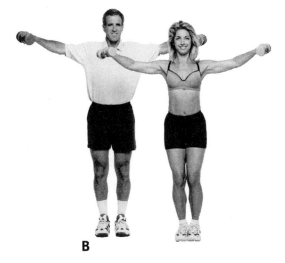

B

Start with the Triceps Kickbacks; as you develop your upper body, switch to the more challenging Triceps Dips.

Triceps Kickbacks

The triceps are one of the most underused muscle groups of the body; we primarily use our biceps (front of arms) in our daily chores, such as lifting groceries or a baby. Hold a weight in both hands, with legs shoulder-width apart and slightly bent [A]. Keeping your abs tight and your back flat, bend your elbows so your upper arms are almost parallel to the floor, elbows in close to your body [B]. Squeeze the backs of your arms as you straighten

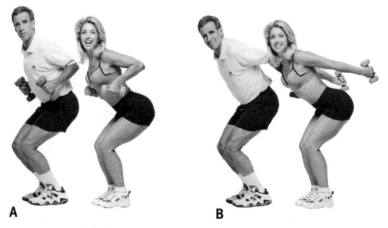

A   B

your arms to lift the weights directly behind you. Then bend
elbows to bring weights back to your sides. *Benefits: Strengthens
backs of arms (triceps). No more sagging arms!*

Triceps Dips (Advanced)

Place your hands on the edge of a sturdy bench or chair, fingers
facing forward, knees bent at 90-degree angles [A]. Keeping
your buttocks in close to the bench, bend your elbows to slowly
lower yourself toward the floor, until your elbows are bent at
close to 90-degree angles [B]. Squeeze your triceps as you
straighten arms to return to starting position, then repeat.
Benefits: Strengthens backs of arms (triceps).

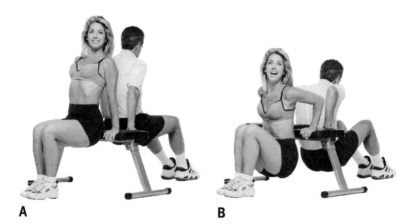

A   B

Abs /Lower Back

Do one set of 15 to 20 repetitions for each of the next four moves. After you complete all four moves (which should take about three to five minutes), repeat the entire circuit again.

Reverse Crunch

Lie on your back with one knee bent at a 90-degree angle and the other leg extended up straight in the air, feet flexed, hands behind your head. Keeping your back flat on the floor, exhale as you use your lower abdominal muscles to gently lift your hips off the floor, pressing your belly button in toward your spine. Pull your knee in as close to your chest as possible; the other leg stays straight and extended in the air. This is a very small movement; your knee should stay bent at the same angle throughout the move. Try to control the lift using your abdominal muscles—don't rely on momentum! Inhale as you release. Relax and repeat with other leg. Alternate legs for a total of 15 to 20 reps. *Benefits: Strengthens lower abdominals.*

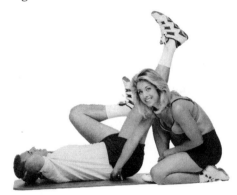

Basic Crunch

Lie on your back with your knees bent and your feet flat on the floor. If you're a beginner or have neck problems, place a pillow or a rolled-up towel under your neck and head for support. Press your lower back firmly into the floor; there shouldn't be an arch in your back at all. Rest your head in your hands—or cross your arms in front of your chest (see photo) for an extra challenge—keeping your neck and shoulders relaxed. Exhale as you tighten your abdominals and slowly lift your shoulders off the floor, keeping your abs contracted. Inhale as you slowly

Ward off middle-age spread with ▼ crunches!

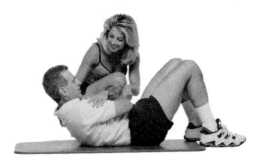

lower your shoulders back to the floor and repeat. *Benefits:
Strengthens entire rectus abdominus—a complete ab exercise!*

Bicycles

Lie on your back with your legs extended straight up in the air.
Press your back firmly into the floor—there should be no arch
in your back. Rest your head in your hands, but make sure your
neck and shoulders are relaxed. Keeping your left leg straight
and suspended, pull your right knee into your chest as you
reach your left shoulder blade toward your right knee.
Straighten your right leg and return your left shoulder to the
floor, then repeat on the opposite side, pulling your left knee in
toward your chest and lifting your right shoulder. Be sure to lift
with your abdominal muscles—don't pull on your neck with
your arms. Continue alternating sides for all reps. *Benefits:
Strengthens upper and lower abs (rectus abdominus) and
obliques (sides of waist).*

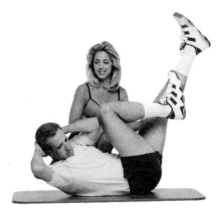

Stretches

You've tested and really worked your muscles today—so reward yourself with the following stretches. They're a great way to end your workout! You can do this on your own or with a partner.

Saddle Stretch

Sit on the floor. Place your feet apart and gently keep your legs straight. Place your hands on the floor and slowly pull yourself forward until you feel an easy stretch in your groin. Make sure you bend from the hips and not from your shoulders. Hold the stretch for 15 to 20 seconds. *Benefits: Stretches inner thighs, groin area and hips.*

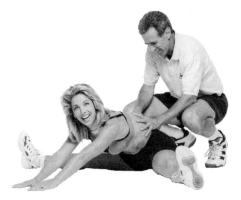

Hamstring Stretch

Lie on your back on the floor with your knees bent and your feet on the floor. Raise your right leg up and pull it toward your chest. You can use a towel to assist you. Hold the stretch for 15 to 20 seconds. Lower your leg and repeat the stretch with your left leg. To feel a greater stretch in the calf muscle, wrap the

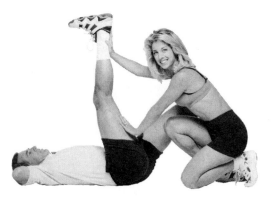

towel around the ball of the foot. *Benefits: Stretches hamstrings (backs of thighs)—important for a healthy lower back!*

Upper-Body Stretch

Sit on the floor. Place your hands behind your neck. Slowly press your elbows slightly back. Hold for 15 to 20 seconds. Relax and repeat. *Benefits: Great for posture. Increases flexibility in the upper body; especially opens up the chest (pectoral muscles).*

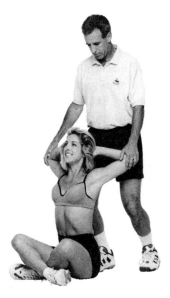

10

Wednesday: Fat-Burning Blast

Are you ready to whittle away fat and accelerate your calorie-burning ability? This fast-paced 30-minute circuit combines fat-blasting cardiovascular exercises with muscle-building weight-training moves for a major metabolic boost. In other words, you not only burn fat during the workout, but you continue burning it at a significantly elevated rate after you stop, whether you're sitting at your desk or sleeping.

Here's what to expect on Wednesdays: After a short cardio warm-up (important for getting your muscles ready for action), you'll do one minute of body sculpting followed by two minutes of aerobic exercise. For the next 30 minutes, you'll continue this sequence for a total-body blast! At the end, take five more minutes to do the ab exercises and stretches pictured on pages 173 to 176.

So get your weights ready—you'll need 3- to 5-pound weights. (Since you'll be sustaining each body-sculpting move for one minute and will have the added challenge of moving your feet, stick to lighter weights, even if you used heavier ones during Tuesday's weight-training workout.) Put them within reach, but not where you may trip over them. Since music is a great motivator, turn on your favorite tunes and get set to move. If you prefer to follow along with a video, try my new series that complements this book or my *Power Kickboxing* or *Fat-Burning Blast* tapes.

Remember: If you already have a favorite aerobic workout, feel free to stick with it. Or, for other super cardio options, check out the list on page 15. But after your 20 to 30 minutes of cardio, be sure to do the body-sculpting exercises pictured on the following pages to develop those muscles. Do two 12- to 15-rep sets of biceps curls, overhead presses, triceps toners, upright rows, lower-tummy tighteners and waistline slimmers. Finish your workout with the stretches shown on pages 175 to 176.

Instructions: Repeat the following sequence twice.

WARM-UP
March in place
3 minutes
Advanced: Run in place

BODY SCULPTING
Biceps Curls with Heel Taps
1 minute
Hold a 3- or 5-pound weight in each hand with an underhand grip. Alternate heel taps (touching your heel to the floor in front of you) as you bend both elbows to raise the weights toward your shoulders, keeping your elbows in close to your body. *Benefits: Strengthens fronts of arms (biceps).* At the end of this move, keep your head above your heart as you return weights to the floor.

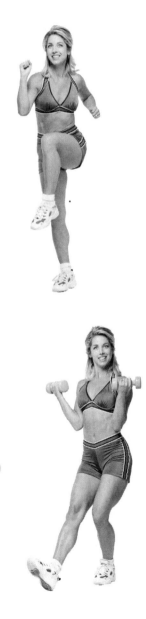

CARDIO
Crossovers
2 minutes

With your hands behind your head, tighten your abdominals as you raise your left knee to touch your right elbow. Concentrate on lifting your knee, not lowering your elbow. Repeat, raising right knee to left elbow; each crossover should take about 1 to 2 seconds. Keep your abs pulled in as you continue alternating sides for 2 minutes.

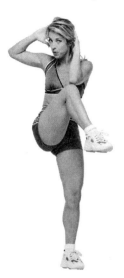

BODY SCULPTING
Overhead Presses with Heel Taps
1 minute

Holding a 3- or 5-pound weight in each hand at shoulder height, raise the weights up over your head; your arms are slightly in front of your body (you should be able to see them out of the corners of your eyes). Alternate heel taps as you lift and lower. *Benefits: Strengthens shoulders, backs of arms (triceps).* At the end of this move, keep your head above your heart as you return weights to the floor.

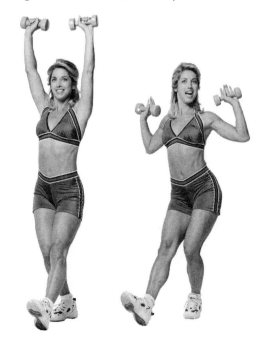

CARDIO
"Kickboxing"
Front Kicks
2 minutes

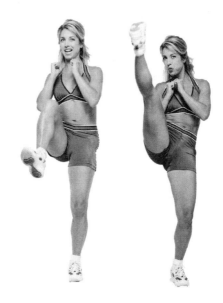

To begin, start in the guard position: feet hip-width apart, one foot slightly in front of the other, hands in loose fists in front of your chin, palms facing each other. Tighten your abs as you lift your knee to waist height, then "kick" your lower leg forward toward your "target"; for balance, your upper body leans back slightly as you kick. Return leg to starting position and repeat kicks with the same leg for 1 minute. Switch legs and repeat. Keep your arms in guard position as you alternate kicks. These kicks are challenging; if you need to take a break, march in place—don't stop entirely.

BODY SCULPTING
Triceps Toners while
marching in place
1 minute

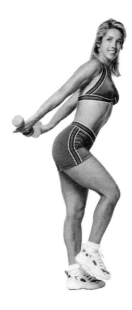

Holding a 3- or 5-pound weight in each hand, march in place as you do triceps toners: Extend both elbows behind you, elbows in close to your body (like in a Triceps Kick-back). Squeeze the backs of your arms as you straighten your arms to lift the weights directly behind you. Continue lifting and lowering weights behind you. *Benefits: Strengthens backs of arms (triceps).* At the end of this move, keep your head above your heart as you return weights to the floor.

CARDIO
Punches
2 minutes

Begin your punching sequence in guard position: feet hip-width apart, one foot slightly in front of the other, hands in loose fists in front of your chin, palms facing each other. If you're throwing punches with your right arm, your left foot should be in front; if you're throwing with your left, your right foot is forward. Lean your body weight into each punch; once you have the punches down, pick up the pace to turn up the burn!

Jab

Tighten your abs and bend both your knees as you throw this basic forward punch into your imaginary opponent's chin. Keep your muscles flexed and firm; don't lock your elbows. Do 20 jabs with each arm.

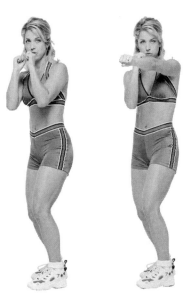

Hook

With the hook punch, your fist moves in a semicircular motion around and into the side of your "opponent's" jaw. Keep your arm bent and parallel to the floor. Tighten your abs and bend your knees as you punch. Do 20 hooks with each arm.

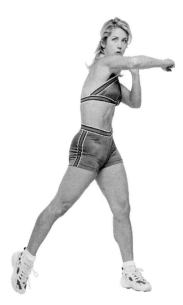

Uppercut

With the uppercut, your fist moves in a semicircle from below your hip up into your "opponent's" chin. Keep your elbow in close to your body, tighten your abs and bend your knees as you punch. Do 20 uppercuts with each arm.

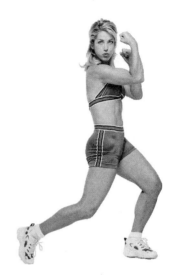

BODY SCULPTING
Upright Rows while marching in place
1 minute

Hold 3- or 5-pound dumbbells in front of you, palms facing toward you. Squeeze your shoulder blades together as you raise the weights to chin height, elbows bent out to the side. March in place as you lift and lower. *Benefits: Strengthens upper back.* At the end of this move, keep your head above your heart as you return weights to the floor.

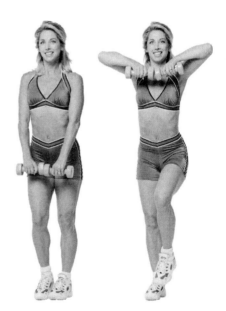

CARDIO
"Kickboxing" Back Kicks
2 minutes

Start in guard position: feet hip-width apart, one foot slightly in front of the other, hands in loose fists in front of your chin, palms facing each other. Tighten your abs as you sit back into a squat. Raise one knee and kick your leg back behind you, like a donkey kick. Look back over your shoulder at your "opponent" as you kick. Do 20 kicks, then switch legs and repeat. Continue switching legs until your 2 minutes are up. These kicks are challenging; if you need to take a break, march in place—don't stop entirely.

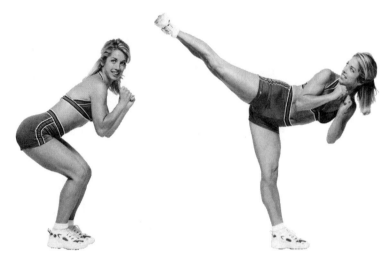

Ab Firmers

Lower-Tummy Tightener

Lie on your back with your knees bent and lifted so they're above your hips and the soles of your feet together. Keep your back flat on the floor as you use your lower abs to lift your feet 6 to 8 inches, pressing the small of the back against the floor. Keep your abs tight as you lower and repeat. This is a very short range of movement: The focus here is pressing your belly button in and your lower back into the floor. Do two sets of 12 to 15 reps. *Benefits: Strengthens lower abs.*

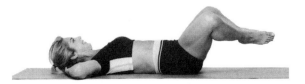

Waistline Slimmer

Sit on the floor with your knees bent in front of you, feet tucked to the right side; place your hands on the floor directly under your shoulders for support, elbows slightly bent. Contract the muscles on the sides of your waist as you lift up your knees and shift them to the left, moving your feet to the right. Be sure to keep your elbows bent and lean slightly back to take the pressure off your back. Alternate sides for 15 to 20 reps. *Benefits: Strengthens obliques (sides of the waistline).*

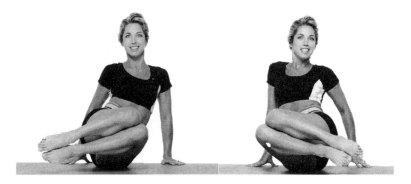

Reciprocal Reach

Lie on your belly with your arms and legs extended and your feet about 6 inches apart. Slowly raise your head and left arm about 4 to 6 inches from the floor as you squeeze your buttocks and lift your right leg about 4 to 8 inches from the floor. Look down at the floor to keep your neck in alignment and anchor your hips to the floor. Concentrate on proper from—do not overarch your back. Hold for 10 seconds, then release. Switch sides and repeat. Continue alternating sides for all reps. *Benefits: Strengthens lower back and spine.*

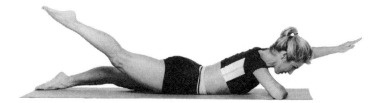

Stretches

Wall Hang
Stand an arm's distance away
from a wall; lean over and
place your hands on the wall
just above your head. Step
back about 2 feet. Keeping
your legs straight (don't
lock your knees), extend
through your back as you
press your hips back and chest
down. Hold for 20 seconds.
*Benefits: Stretches back and
hamstrings.*

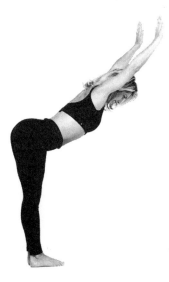

Wall Squat
Stand with your back against a wall. Step forward with both
feet so only your back is resting against the wall. Slowly slide
your back down the wall until you're in a squatting position.
(Modification: Skip the wall slide and start by squatting with
your back flat against the wall, feet in close to your buttocks.)
Hold your arms out straight in front of you. Inhale and exhale
deeply as you hold for 20 seconds, keeping your back as
straight as possible. *Benefits: Stretches lower back, hips,
buttocks and Achilles tendons.*

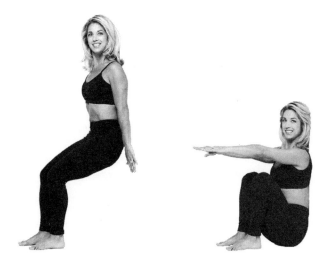

Butterfly

Facing a wall, lie on your back, arms by your sides. Place a pillow or rolled towel under your head (optional). Slide your buttocks up against a wall. Open and relax your knees, letting
them fall out to the sides, and place the soles of your feet
together. Hold for 20 seconds. *Benefits: Stretches hips and legs.*

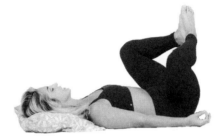

11

Thursday: Toning with Yoga and Pilates Method

I've been in the fitness industry for more than 20 years. For much of that time, I mainly focused on aerobics and weight training. Then, about seven years ago, I fell in love with yoga—it balances out my high-impact workouts and builds strong, flexible muscles. And lately, I've started doing Pilates Method exercises because they help give my body a longer, leaner look. While I still love to run and lift weights, these softer, more spiritual workouts help create a balanced body from the inside out.

Discover the beauty of yoga and Pilates: renewed energy, better concentration, peace of mind, and a balanced body from the inside out.

In theory, these two workouts are very different. Yoga is a centuries-old tradition rooted in Hindu and Buddhist cultures that not only helps build a strong, healthy body but teaches more spiritual breathing and meditation techniques. Pilates, on the other hand, was developed in the early 1900s by a man named Joseph Pilates (pronounced puh-LAH-tees) who trained professional dancers. With both, you develop strength, flexibility and balance by moving your muscles through a series of controlled move-ments, or "poses."

I started doing exercises like these at age 12 as part of my gym-nastics training. V-sits, single-leg reaches, leg pulls and T-stands are the kinds of moves that prepare you to do hip-ups on the uneven bars and back walkovers on the balance beam. But they also help you on a day-to-day basis by conditioning your muscles in a balanced way and increasing your self-awareness by drawing your focus inward.

I've borrowed some of the fundamentals from these two pow-erful workouts and created a fantastic total-body sculpting rou-tine, pictured on the following pages. These soft, fluid exercises condition your body without punishing it. After weight training, it's a refreshing new approach to toning!

In the routine, you'll begin with some wonderful yoga stand-ing postures designed to warm up your body and improve your balance. Then you'll do a series of Pilates-based moves to tone your waistline, your abs and your torso and increase your flexi-blity. Finally, we'll cool down with a few seated yoga poses that also promote strong, supple muscles and balance.

While the exercises on these pages may look easy, you'll quickly see how much strength it takes to hold your body in these differ-ent positions. As you do each move, focus on maintaining proper form and alignment; don't sacrifice technique to save a few sec-onds. Your movements should be smooth and controlled. If you have trouble with a pose, don't get frustrated—keep practicing, and soon you'll develop the strength needed to do it correctly.

It's important to remember that every one of these moves orig-inates at your core—that is, your belly or your abs. Be sure to keep your tummy tight throughout each pose. If you lose your balance, tighten those abs—it will help place your body into proper alignment. You should also focus on elongating your spine as you go from one pose to the next; this will help keep your spine flexible and healthy.

As you move through the poses, use your breath to draw your mind into the present and whisk the tension out of your body. In yoga, your goal is to breathe in and out through the nose. It's not easy to do, but the more you practice, the more natural it will feel. In Pilates Method, you'll inhale deeply through your nose as you enter a pose and exhale through your mouth as you release the pose. Notice your chest and belly expand as you draw air into your body's core, and fill your entire body with energy-giving oxygen.

You can also use your mind to maintain your balance, as some of these poses can feel a bit awkward at first. For standing postures, focus on one item directly in front of you—a lamp, a light switch, a wall hanging. Whenever you start to wobble or fall over, remember to stare at your focal point. If you lose your concentration, you'll be more likely to topple!

One of the best things about yoga and Pilates-inspired moves is that they offer numerous benefits for your emotional health as well. As you move through the exercises, observe how your body feels and try to release any built-up stress that you may be harboring. Are you clenching your jaw? Tensing your shoulders? This routine is designed to have a calming effect—the smooth, steady movements quiet your mind and soothe your nervous system. Focus on letting the tension go, and you'll be on the path to a healthier body both inside and out.

If you enjoy these moves, try my *Fit and Lite* show on Lifetime—Television for Women. It's a great combination of yoga, Pilates-inspired exercises and my "Denise's Daily Wisdoms" to help get you through your busy life!

DENISEOLOGY
It's often said, "You're as young as your spine."
Your spine is your lifeline. So keep your back healthy!

Yoga and Pilates Method Toning Workout

As you learn each move and become more practiced, try to flow from one to the next without stopping. Maintain constant awareness of your breath; let the flow of oxygen in and out of your body work for you. Unless otherwise instructed, do each move one time. Do each move slowly—there's no rush! If you lose your balance or have trouble with a pose, keep working at it until you feel comfortable. If there's a lot of time remaining at the end of the Pilates Method, do some of the moves again before doing the Yoga Cool-Down and Meditation.

Some of these exercises have been designated beginner, intermediate or advanced. If you've never done yoga or the Pilates Method before, start with the beginner moves and, over the next few weeks, experiment with the intermediate and advanced moves. My goal is to have you challenge yourself. You'll be amazed by what your body can do when you try! If you *have* tried yoga and Pilates Method before, do the intermediate and advanced moves; for variety, occasionally throw in one or two beginner moves, too.

Yoga

Warrior I (Beginner)

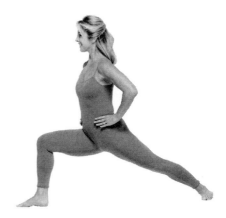

Stand with your hands on your hips; step your feet apart so your ankles are in line with your wrists (your feet will be about 3 to 4 feet apart). Turn your left foot out at a 90-degree angle so your toes point directly to the left and rotate your right foot so your toes point to the left at a 45-degree angle. Bend your left knee as close as you can to a 90-degree angle (knee is directly over your ankle). Keeping your right leg straight, rotate your upper body so you're facing left. Push into your right heel. Look straight ahead or upward slightly. Take three deep, nourishing breaths, inhaling and exhaling through your nose. Return to starting position and repeat on opposite side.

Warrior II (Intermediate)

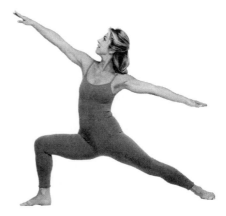

Start in same position as Warrior I, with your left knee bent at a 90-degree angle, your arms extended to the front and the back. Keeping your shoulders relaxed, hold pose for two or three deep breaths. Feel proud in this warrior position. Return to starting position and repeat on opposite side.

Warrior III (Advanced)

From Warrior II, extend both arms over your head, palms facing each other and fingers pointing toward the ceiling. Focus your eyes on your hands. Hold pose for two breaths. Return to starting position and repeat on the other side.

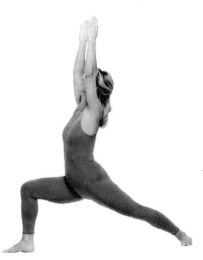

Modified Triangle Level I (Beginner)

Stand with your legs 3 or 4 feet apart. Extend arms straight out to the sides at shoulder height, palms facing down. Turn your left foot out, away from your body, as in first position in ballet. Keeping your right leg straight, bend your left leg, resting your left arm on your left thigh for support. If you're flexible enough, place your left hand on your left calf or foot. To give your neck a good stretch, turn your head to look at the ceiling. Take two deep breaths. Return to starting position and repeat on opposite side.

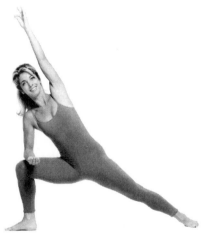

Triangle Level II (Intermediate)

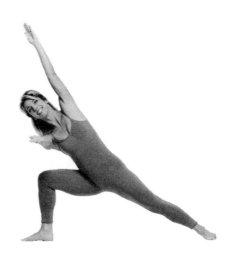

Stand with your legs 3 or 4 feet apart. Extend your arms straight out to the sides at shoulder height, palms facing down. Turn your left foot out, away from your body, as in first position in ballet. Keeping one leg straight, bend your torso to the left, resting your left arm on your thigh, as in Level I. When you're ready, take your left arm off your left thigh and extend it straight in front of you, palm facing up. This may seem like the Level I pose, but it isn't . . . you'll feel it in your waistline and be working different muscles. Take two deep breaths. Return to starting position and repeat on opposite side.

Triangle Level with a Twist

Stand with your feet about 3 feet apart, with your feet pointing forward. Bend forward, reaching your right arm toward the floor and reaching your left arm straight up over your head. Hold the position and take three deep breaths. Slowly come back up to a standing position and repeat on the other side.

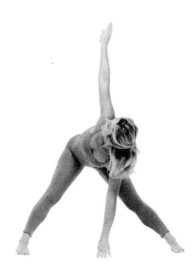

Tree Pose

If you're a beginner, you may want to use a chair or a wall to help maintain your balance. Stand with your feet together and your arms hanging loosely by your sides, palms facing in toward you. Allow an imaginary string to pull your head up, lengthening your spine; tighten your thigh muscles, but keep your shoulders and hands relaxed. Raise your left knee until your foot is about even with your right knee. Rotate your left knee out to the left and rest the sole of your left foot on the inner thigh of your right leg, as high as possible. Place your palms together at chest level—a prayerlike position. Keeping your palms together, raise your arms over your head. Take three deep breaths. Return to starting position and repeat on opposite side.

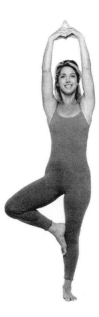

Spinal Twist

Sit on the floor with your legs extended in front of you, feet flexed. Bend your left knee, then lift your left foot up and place it on the opposite side of your right knee. Turn your upper body to the left. Bending your right arm, place your right elbow on the outside of your left knee. Try to keep your shoulders down as you twist your spine farther to the left. Pushing your chest forward will further lengthen your spine. Hold the pose for three deep breaths. Return to starting position and repeat on opposite side.

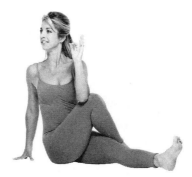

Child's Pose

Start in an upright kneeling position. Sit back on your heels. Keeping your buttocks down on your heels, slowly bend forward and lower your head to the floor until you're curled up like a sleeping child, your forehead resting on the floor, arms extended in front of you, palms facing down. Take five deep breaths—and relax! This pose is designed to rejuvenate and nurture.

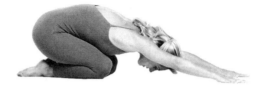

Pilates Method

The Hundred (Beginner)

Lie on your back, then pull your knees into your chest and place your arms over your head. Gently pull your chin forward to lift your head, neck and shoulder blades off the floor. Move arms in a semicircle out to your sides and then down so your fingers are reaching toward your toes. Lift your arms 2 to 3 inches off the floor, then quickly pump (or pulse) your arms up and down. Breathe—inhale for five counts and exhale for five counts. Do this five times.

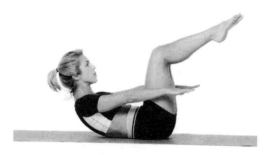

The Hundred (Advanced)

Same as above, but extend your legs straight up into the air and then lower them to the floor as much as possible while keeping your spine pressed against the floor and your belly flat. Hold this pose while you count to 100.

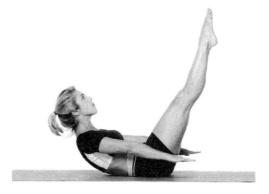

Leg Pull — Back Support

Sit on the floor with your legs straight out in front of you, feet together. Lift your hands by your sides, palms down and fingers facing back. Press your hips up to create a straight line from the crown of your head to your toes. Look forward. Keep your belly flat. Without shifting your weight, inhale as you lift your left leg, then exhale as you lower it back down to the floor. Repeat with your right leg. Continue alternating legs until you've done three to six lifts with each leg.

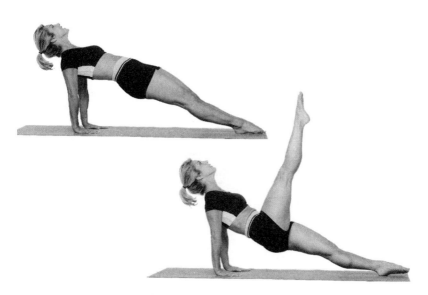

Leg Pull—Front Support

Lie on your belly. Flex your feet and lift yourself into a push-up position, creating a long line from your head to your heels. Keeping your abs and buttocks tight, lift your left leg and lower. Try not to shift your weight as you lift. Keep your torso still. Return to starting position, then repeat with your right leg. Do four times on each side. Don't forget to breathe!

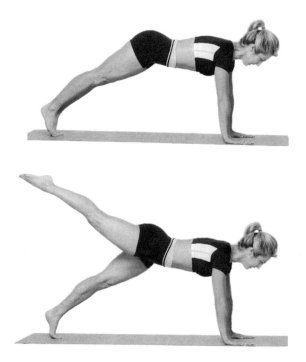

Twist T-Stand

Sit on your right hip with your legs slightly bent and your right hand on the floor directly under your shoulder. Pushing up on your right hand, inhale as you lift your hips off the floor and straighten your legs to create a straight line from your head to your toes, keeping your abs and buttocks tight and your shoulders relaxed. Lift your left arm up over your head to form the letter T. Hold for 10 to 15 seconds. Exhale as you lower your hips and bring your left arm back down to your side. Do three times, then switch sides and repeat.

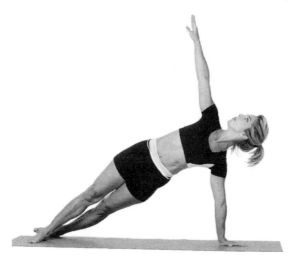

Single Leg Reach (Scissors)

This ab exercise is a little more difficult because it involves most of the abdominal region. Concentrate on keeping your belly button pulled in and your back pressed into the floor. Lie on the floor with one leg straight and the other knee bent toward your chest. Using your abdominal muscles, lift your feet and shoulders off the floor. Then slowly raise your right leg as high as you can, while keeping the left leg just above the floor. Exhale as you switch legs, and continue to alternate legs with smooth, controlled motions for 8 to 12 reps. Relax and repeat.

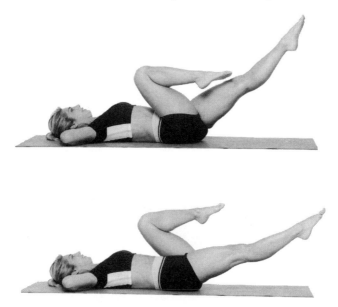

Criss-Cross (Bicycles)

Lie on your back. Pull your knees into your chest and extend your arms over your head. Pull your chin forward. Rest your head in your hands. Lift your upper body (your head, neck and shoulders) off the floor. Exhale as you extend your right leg out straight while twisting your left elbow toward your left knee. Inhale as you return to center with both knees bent toward your chest. Repeat, this time extending your left leg out straight and twisting with your right elbow. Continue alternating legs 12 times total.

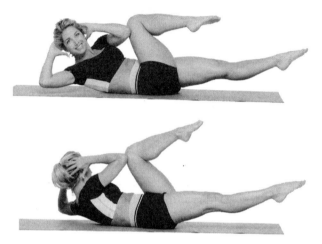

Flat Back

Kneel down on all fours, with your hands directly under your shoulders and with your back flat. Keeping your abdominals tight, inhale as you extend your left leg behind you and your right arm in front of you until they're both parallel to the floor. Hold for 10 to 15 seconds, making sure you pull in your abs and contract them. Exhale as you return your legs and arms to starting position (kneeling on all fours). Repeat, this time extending your right leg and left arm. Continue alternating sides three times total on each side. This is one of the best exercises to strengthen the muscles that align your spine to keep your back healthy.

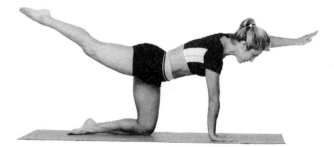

Pelvic Curl

Lie on your back with your knees bent, feet flat on the floor. Maintain a line with your neck and shoulders relaxed. Inhale as you use your abdominal muscles to slowly lift your hips up off the floor. Continue curling (lifting) until your ribs, hipbones and knees are in one line (see photo), reaching the knees up and away. Hold for 5 seconds, then exhale as you lower your spine one vertebra at a time. Repeat three times—and take your time!

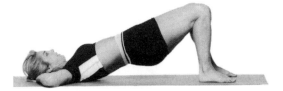

The Roll-Up

Slowly roll your body up and forward, tightening your abdominal muscles. Now, slowly roll back, feeling and massaging each vertebra and pressing your back into the mat. Focus on your lower abs, below your belly button. Try to keep your feet off the floor throughout the movement. Rock slightly forward and backward, about 8 to 12 times.

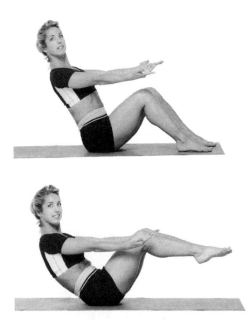

Teaser—V-sit (Advanced)

Lie on the floor on your back with your legs straight and your arms extended overhead. Inhale as you lift both legs while raising both arms overhead and in front of you until your fingers are pointed toward your toes. Your entire body should form a V, with your weight balanced on your buttocks. Keep your legs extended in the air as you exhale and slowly roll your upper body back down to the floor, vertebra by vertebra, and return your arms to the overhead position. Repeat three times.

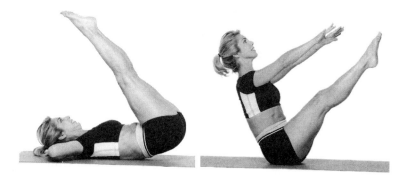

Swimming

Lie on your belly with your legs straight, feet hip-width apart and slightly turned out, and your arms extended out straight over your head, palms facing down. Place your body weight over your pelvis and lower ribs, press your belly button toward your spine and elongate your neck, keeping your shoulders down and relaxed. Inhale as you simultaneously lift your right arm and your left leg a few inches off the floor. Exhale as you lower and repeat, this time lifting your left arm and right leg. Continue switching sides for 12 reps total, gradually picking up your pace. Do a total of three 12-rep sets. Be sure to squeeze your buttocks muscles so you won't over-arch your lower back.

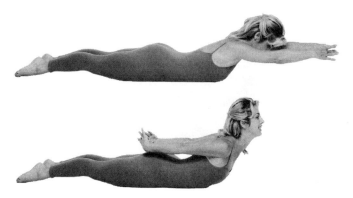

Yoga Cool-Down

Cat Stretch

This is a great way to strengthen your abs as well as keep your back flexible. Kneel on all fours, being careful not to let your stomach sag. Inhale as you keep your back flat, chin and chest lifted slightly upward [A]. Now, exhale as you slowly roll up your back, pull in your belly button and tighten your abdominal muscles [B]. Do three complete sequences, inhaling and exhaling.

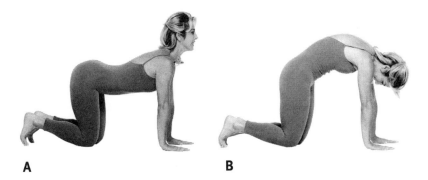

A   **B**

Downward Dog

I like to begin this pose from a kneeling position. Or you can flow directly into this pose from the Cat Stretch. Kneel on all fours. Push up using your arm muscles as you lift your hips and buttocks up toward the ceiling, straightening your legs. Feel as though you're pointing your tailbone up toward the ceiling to form a triangle. Now try to slowly and gently press your heels down, feeling the stretch in your calves. Hold the pose, as shown, for three deep breaths. Relax and repeat twice.

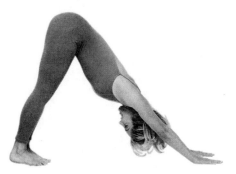

Bridge/Camel (Advanced)

Lie on your back with your knees bent, feet flat on the floor, hip-width apart (your knees are directly above your ankles). Place your arms by your sides. Walk your heels in close to your buttocks and lift your hips up, supporting your lower back with both hands; your upper arms, shoulders, neck and head remain on the floor. Squeeze your buttocks together. Take three deep breaths, then lower to starting position.

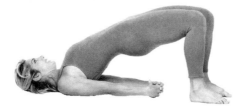

Meditation

• Set an egg timer for 5 or 10 minutes (depending on how much time you have).

• Make sure your space is quiet and free from distractions such as phone calls or television.

• Lie on your back with your arms at your sides and your legs slightly apart. If your back bothers you, place a pillow under your knees. Allow your body to relax and "fall" into the floor. There should be no tension in your limbs.

• Clear your mind of all thoughts. This isn't easy—I know. We are all so busy that our minds race constantly. But try to keep your mind in the moment for the next 10 minutes. Concentrate on your breathing and relaxing every part of your body. If your mind returns to thoughts of your grocery list, push them aside by breathing deeply. You have the power to control your thoughts. Do it!

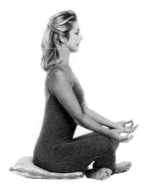

• When the egg timer sounds, slowly roll to your right side before pushing yourself upright and then sitting in a seated, cross-legged pose. Take three deep, cleansing breaths. As you exhale, release all the stress from your body.

12 | Friday: Circuit Training

Ready to ignite your metabolism? You're *really* going to burn butter now!

Circuit training may be new to you, but it's been around since the 1950s. What is it exactly? A "circuit" is a series of exercises done one after the next without stopping. The goal is to move quickly from one to the next to keep your heart rate elevated—and burn, burn, burn those calories!

There are different kinds of circuit-training workouts. You can do purely aerobic or strength-training circuits. Or you can mix cardiovascular and strength-building moves, as we're going to do during today's workout. This is a time-efficient routine—you score both aerobic and body-sculpting workouts in just 30 minutes. A total-body blast!

This fast-paced workout does call for a bit of equipment—but if you don't have it all, you can substitute items that you have around the house:

> 3-, 5-, and 8-pound weights (substitute: soup cans or water bottles)
> Jump rope (substitute: simulated jump rope)
> Weight bench (substitute: a sturdy chair with a straight back)

When I circuit train, I either go into my little home gym or push my family-room furniture aside and create three different stations. I put a jump rope in one station, a set of dumbbells in another and an exercise mat in the third. I put on my favorite music to get me motivated and, for the next 30 minutes, I move from station to station. In a flash, my workout is over!

How much weight should you use? Start with 3-pound dumbbells or soup cans. At the end of a move (15 to 20 reps), if your muscles don't feel challenged, it's time to switch to the next weight increment—maybe two pounds heavier. As you build strength over the next four weeks, you might want to keep readjusting your weights so your progress continues.

So get your jump rope and weights ready—and prepare for action! You don't need to rearrange your living room; just clear enough space so you won't trip over your rope or dumbbells. For the next 30 minutes, I want you to move constantly. If you get tired, don't stop; simply march in place. Put 110 percent into this end-of-the-week workout! You can do it!

Remember: If you already have a favorite aerobic workout, feel free to stick with it. Or you can pick from a list of supercharged cardio workouts on page 15. But after your 20 to 30 minutes of cardio, be sure to do the strength moves pictured on the following pages to work your muscles. Do two 12- to 15-rep sets of incline chest presses, torso trimmers, one-arm rows, extended crunches, upper-back firmers, low hovers and oblique toners. Finish your workout with the stretches shown on pages 201 to 202.

Do all of the following exercises in this order. Try not to rest between exercises; if you get tired, simply march in place; as soon as you feel ready, pick up the exercise again. After you've completed all the exercises listed here, repeat the entire circuit. Don't forget to leave a few minutes to do the stretches at the end.

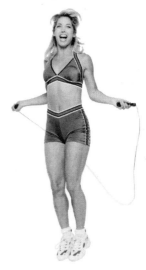

Cardio
Jump Rope
3 minutes
Once you master basic jumping rope, try variations, such as alternating heel taps (touching your heels to the floor in front of you) while you jump or quick skipping (like a boxer). If you don't have a rope, just pretend you have one.

STRENGTH
Incline Chest Press
1 minute

If you don't have an incline weight bench, lie on the floor with two big pillows under your back to prop yourself up; during the exercise, your elbows will be lower than the surface of your back. Lie on your back with elbows out to the sides, then straighten your arms, pressing the weights straight up into the air. Do about 15 to 20 reps or until you can't do another one. If you finish early, march in place until the minute is up. At the end of this move, keep your head above your heart as you return weights to the floor.

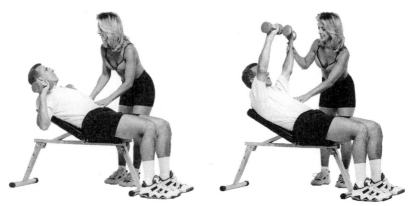

STRENGTH
Torso Trimmer
1 minute

Lie on your side; prop yourself up on your elbow, your elbow directly beneath your shoulder. Extend your legs out to your side as pictured. Place your hand behind your head. Slowly crunch forward,

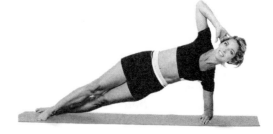

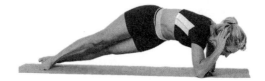

touching your elbow in front of your fingertips. Come back up to starting position. Do three to five times, then switch sides and repeat. This is challenging, so take your time. This move is excellent for the sides of your waistline.

CARDIO
Squat Jumps
2 minutes

Stand with your feet together, your arms by your sides. Sit back into a squat, keeping your back straight and your abs pulled in; your thighs should be as close to parallel to the floor as possible. From the squat, jump into the air, reaching your arms toward the ceiling as you jump. Bend your knees when you land to minimize the impact. Repeat.

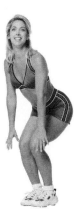
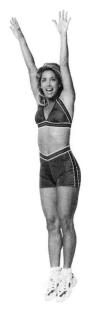

STRENGTH
One-Arm Rows
1 minute

Stand with your feet apart as shown. Bend your knees slightly and keep your abs tight. Rest your palm on your front thigh or use a chair for support. Begin with your arm extended all the way down so you get a good stretch. Keeping your back flat (not rounded), slowly lift the weight up toward your armpit. Slowly lower and repeat 15 times and then switch sides.

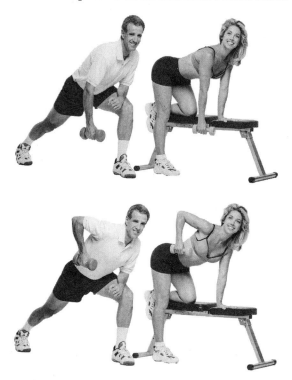

STRENGTH
Extended Crunches
1 minute

Lie on your back with your feet elevated straight up. Contract your abs as you reach your fingertips toward your toes; your head, neck and shoulders lift off the floor. Keeping your head lifted, pulse up and down 15 to 20 times. Rest for 15 seconds, relaxing your neck and placing your head on the floor,

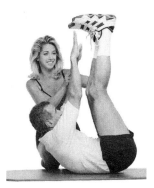

then do another set of 15 to 20 reaches. If you're a beginner or you aren't as flexible, bend your knees and do the same movement; you'll still get a good workout!

CARDIO
Waist Twists
2 minutes

Think slalom: With your feet together, lightly jump and pivot your knees and toes to the right; simultaneously raise your right elbow out to the right at shoulder height and extend your left arm straight out to the left. Without lowering your arms, repeat on opposite side: Lightly jump and pivot your toes and knees to the left as you bend your left elbow and extend your right arm straight out to the right. Feel the stretch through your waist. Continue alternating sides, gradually picking up the pace.

STRENGTH
Upper-Back Firmers
1 minute

Sit on a chair or bench with your legs out in front of you. Lean forward so that your chest is near your thighs. Holding a dumbbell in each hand, slowly lift your arms straight out to the sides, leading with your pinky fingers. Squeeze your shoulder blades together. Return to starting position and repeat the movement. Make sure each movement is slow and deliberate; try not to swing the weights.

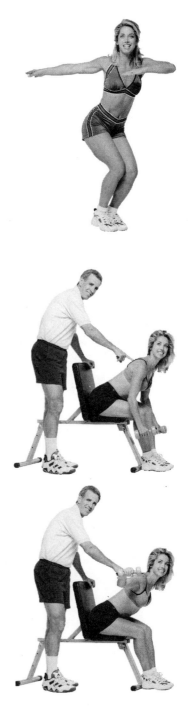

STRENGTH
PART 1
Low Hover
30 seconds

Start in a modified straight-legged push-up position with elbows
on the floor directly below your shoulders, hips lifted slightly,
abdominals tight. Maintaining push-up position from your
elbows, elongate your ab muscles and squeeze buttocks. Hold
for 30 seconds.

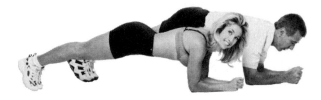

PART 2
Oblique Toners
30 seconds

From the low hover, pull one knee in and reach it toward the
opposite shoulder. Hold for two counts. Return to starting position, then repeat with opposite knee. Focus on keeping abs
pulled in tight. Continue alternating knees for 30 seconds. Take
your time with this one; it's very challenging, but great for the
abs and waistline!

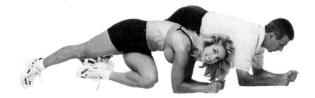

CARDIO
Jack in the Box
2 minutes

With your feet together, squat down as if you're sitting in a chair, then jump up and spread your feet and hands out so your legs and arms both make a V (think jumping jack). Step feet back together, then repeat.

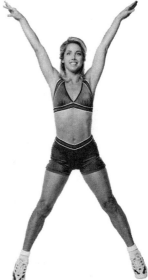

Repeat entire circuit from the beginning.

Stretches

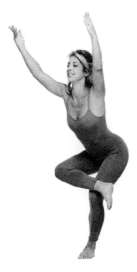

Best Leg Stretch

Stand on your left foot and place your right ankle on your left thigh, your right knee bent out to the side. Bend at the hips slightly and push your buttocks out, reaching both arms up. You can use a chair or wall for balance. *Benefits: Stretches hips, thighs and buttocks.*

Side Stretch

Sit on the floor with your left knee bent, left foot tucked in front of your body, right leg extended straight out to the side. Place your right hand near your right foot as you reach your left arm over your head; hold 20 to 30 seconds, feeling the stretch from your hip all the way up to your fingertips. Switch sides and repeat. *Benefits: Stretches your back and your waist.*

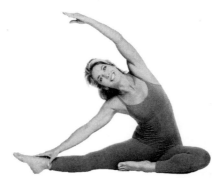

13

Fidget-cize!

DENISEOLOGY

Turn idle time into exercise time! You can tone your muscles whether you're in the kitchen or in front of the TV—no sweat required.

If you're like the hundreds of people who write to me each week, you have trouble finding time to work out. Meetings, errands, laundry, cooking—you're constantly running from one thing to the next. Even when you *want* to work out, you just can't find a free moment—much less a full 30 minutes.

With Fidget-cize, you don't need extra time or even a pair of exercise shoes to get a workout! These mini-workouts can be done anytime, anywhere—whether you're talking on the phone, microwaving your lunch or folding your laundry. Remember: Your muscles don't know whether you're in the gym or in the kitchen. Each exercise takes only a minute (or less) to perform. The goal: to burn calories, lengthen and tone your muscles and learn to move more throughout the day.

When life gets hectic (more often than not), I *really* rely on small movements like these to keep my body limber and strong. While you need 30 minutes of continuous aerobic exercise to keep your heart in tip-top shape, you can stretch and tone your muscles for a minute at a time. Fidget-cize helps get the oxygen flowing to promote good circulation and give you an energy boost—a perfect pick-me-up! Once you incorporate Fidget-cize into your routine, you'll never experience those three o'clock doldrums again.

Believe it or not, you can burn up to 500 calories per day just by fidgeting! Your biggest challenge will be remembering to do them—so post a reminder to yourself in your office or your kitchen. I want this to become as natural as brushing your teeth. Keep practicing, and these calorie-burning movements will soon be a happy, productive habit.

1. Butt and Thigh Toner

Here's a great exercise to firm up your butt and upper thighs. I like to do it when I brush my teeth!

Extend your leg out behind you. Bend your knee with your heel lifting toward your buttocks. Lift and lower your leg. Continue for one full minute. Switch legs and repeat.

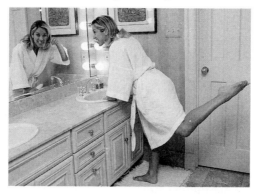

2. Bottoms-Up Squats

This is one of the best thigh exercises that you can do—it's my favorite. You can find me doing it when I ride in an elevator (alone, that is) or when I blow-dry my hair.

Stand with legs hips-width apart. Bend your knees halfway down and back up. Keep going for as long as you can (or until your hair is dry!).

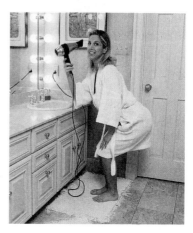

3. Towel Chest Stretch

This easy-does-it stretch leads you to automatic perfect posture. I like to do it just before jumping into the shower.

Stand with your back straight, feet shoulder-width apart, knees slightly bent. Grasp your towel and extend your arms overhead. Press your arms back slowly until you reach a point of tension. Hold for 5 to 10 seconds, then release. Repeat twice.

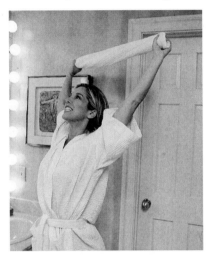

4. Towel Waist Trimmer

You can use your towel for more than just drying off. Why not towel off and trim your waistline at the same time?

Grasp your towel and extend arms overhead. Bend and stretch side to side very slowly, tightening your abs as you stretch. Do 10 waist bends to each side.

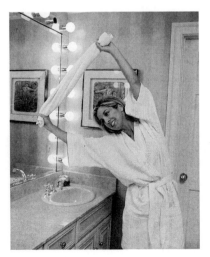

5. Bun Blaster

You'll find me working my buns when I'm cooking, ironing or standing in line.

Stand straight. Lift your right leg straight out behind you, only a few inches off the floor. Point your toes. Squeeze your buttocks tight and feel the muscles tense and work. Keep your hips facing straight ahead and try not to slouch. Return your foot to the floor. Repeat. Don't forget to work both legs!

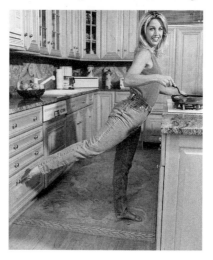

6. Saddlebag Slimmer

You can tone your outer thighs almost anytime, anywhere—diapering the baby, pumping gas or standing at the copy machine.

Stand up tall. Lift your right leg out to the side a few feet, then pull it back in. Repeat 15 times and switch legs.

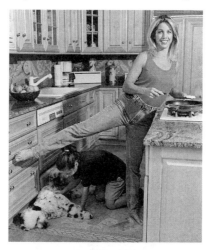

Yes, that's my daughter and my doggie!

7. Inner-Thigh Firmer

This is one of the fastest ways to firm your inner thighs—no more jiggle!

Stand up tall. Pull your right leg in front of your left, gently squeezing your inner thighs. It's a crossover action. Return to the starting position and repeat. Do 15 repetitions before you switch sides.

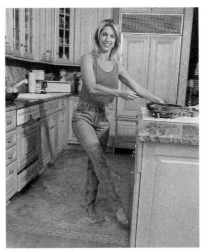

8. Wall Sits

This is my favorite way to make use of phone time!

Lean back lightly against a wall. Flatten your spine against the wall. Lower your body along the wall until your knees are bent to at least a 45-degree angle, but no more than a 90-degree angle. Pretend you are sitting in a chair. Hold for as long as you can—up to 60 seconds.

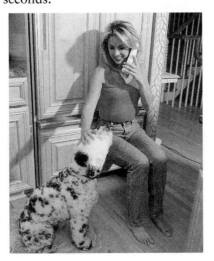

9. Calf Raises

Sculpted calves look sexy in a skirt. Here's a quick way to get them!

Holding on to a banister for balance, place the ball of your right foot on the edge of a step. Press your right heel downward until you feel a stretch in your lower right leg. Hold for 15 to 30 seconds. Lift your heel up so you're on the ball of your foot and hold for 3 seconds. Release. Switch legs and repeat.

10. Triceps Toners

In a hurry, you can quickly shape up the backs of your arms . . . anytime, anywhere.

Holding a paperweight or a can of soup, raise your arm straight above your head. Bend your arm at the elbow and bring the weight down to your shoulder. Your upper arm should remain straight. Repeat 10 times and switch arms.

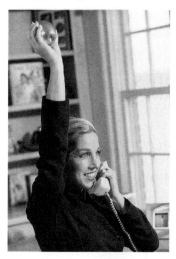

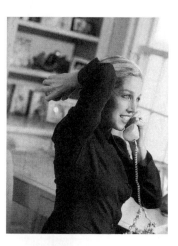

11. Tummy Tuck

I do tummy tucks when sitting on an airplane, in my car, at my desk and while watching TV!

Sit upright in a chair. Hold on to the arms of the chair or a point under the seat of the chair. With your feet together and knees bent, lift your knees toward your chest while contracting your abdominal muscles. Hold for 3 to 5 seconds. Relax and repeat.

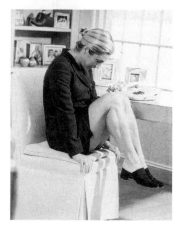

12. Side Stretch

This is a great way to stretch the spine and improve circulation, especially when you've been working at a computer all day.
Interlace your fingers and lift your arms over your head. Press your arms back as far as you can. Slowly lean to the left; hold for 3 to 5 seconds. Then lean to the right and hold for 3 to 5 seconds. Feel the stretch. Don't you feel revitalized?

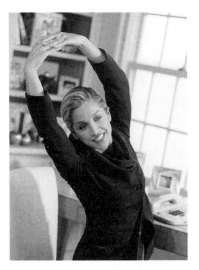

13. Waist Twist— Spine Strengthener

This is a great stretch when you're sitting in front of a computer. I do it while I'm at work or in the car-pool line, waiting for my kids to get out of school.
Sit comfortably, with your back straight. Twist your torso toward the right, far enough that you can grab the back of the seat with both hands. Feel the stretch across your waistline, upper arm and back. Hold for 15 seconds and relax. Twist toward the left.

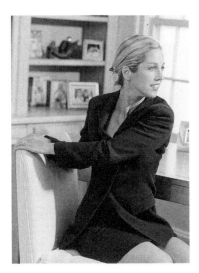

14. Neck Relaxer

Ward off fatigue with this instant neck relaxer.
Sit up straight, with your shoulders relaxed and your neck extended. Lower your left ear slowly to your left shoulder. Hold for 15 seconds. Roll your head to the right and hold your right ear to your right shoulder for 15 seconds. Roll your head to the center. Touch your chin to your chest for 15 seconds. Keeping your chin to your chest, rock your head slowly to the left, then to the right. Semicircle continuously for 15 seconds. Be sure to keep your neck long throughout the entire exercise. Try not to jerk or roll your head backward or in a full circle.

15. Shoulder Rolls

Ever feel like you are carrying the weight of the world on your shoulders? This is a great way to relieve some of that tension! Lift your shoulders to your ears. Inhale. Lower your shoulders and exhale. Repeat. Roll your shoulders up and back five times. Roll your shoulders up and forward five times. Execute three sets of shoulder rolls, backward and forward.

16. Posture Power

Bad posture can cause everything from back pain to a stiff neck. This stretch can help you stand tall by releasing the tension in your back and chest. Clasp your fingers behind your neck. Pull your elbows back as far as you can. Hold for 10 seconds. Keeping your fingers clasped, try to bring your elbows together in front of you. Hold for 5 seconds. Release your hands and relax for 5 seconds. Repeat the sequence three times.

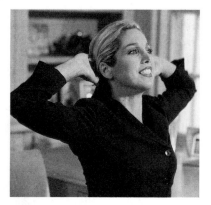

17. Biceps Curls

I work my biceps whether I'm carrying water bottles or my briefcase. Even the stapler on my desk will do for a quick curl! Better yet, keep a set of dumbbells at work—a great mental motivator to keep you working your muscles! Stand with your feet wider than hips-width apart. Your abs should be tight, your back straight and your knees slightly bent. Using an underhand grip, hold the weights in front of your thighs. Exhale as you slowly raise the weights toward your upper arms and shoulders. Hold momentarily and return your hands to the starting position. Keep your shoulders close to your body throughout the movement.

18. Upper-Body Stretch

This great stretch helps open up your chest to ease you into a positive posture and prevent slouching.
Sit up tall. Clasp your hands behind your back. Raise your hands back and up, as high as you can. Hold for 5 to 10 seconds, then release. Repeat twice.

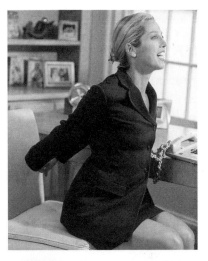

19. Thigh Shaper

Here's a great way to firm the fronts of your thighs, even if you're desk bound. No more flabby knees!
Sit up straight with your feet flat on the floor. Bring one leg out straight in front of you. Maintaining good posture, with your back straight and chin lifted, hold your leg up for 5 to 10 seconds. Lower leg, then repeat with opposite leg. Repeat twice with each leg.

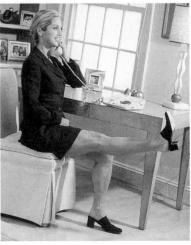

20. Back Relaxer

Here's a wonderful way to relieve the pressure of a tired and achy back. I call it my "knee kiss."
While seated, pull one leg to your chest with both hands and hold for 5 to 10 seconds. Repeat with the opposite leg.

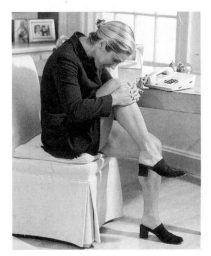

ALMOST INVISIBLE EXERCISES

Muscles can get a workout even without much movement. It's called "isometric" exercise, and it's a godsend in today's push-button society. Here are a few super-subtle moves that you can do whether you're sitting on a bus or sending a fax. No one will suspect a thing!

The Inner-Thigh Squeeze: While sitting, place a tennis ball or your fist between your knees and squeeze your thighs together for 5 to 10 seconds. Feel the tension in your inner thighs!

The Bun Lifter: Squeeze your buttocks muscles for 5 seconds—it's equal to one squat! A super move for your rear view!

The Tummy Tightener: Pull in your tummy, tense and tighten up your ab muscles; hold for 10 seconds. That's equal to one sit-up!

The Seated Ab Firmer: Sit up tall and place your hands on your thighs. Tighten abs as you press your hands against your thighs and pull your knees in toward your chest. Hold for 5 to 10 seconds, then release.

The Triceps Toner: Stand with your arms by your sides, palms facing behind you. Keeping your arms straight, gently pulse your arms backward for 5 seconds, then release. This is a great isometric exercise for the backs of your arms—I do it while waiting in line at the grocery store!

The Arm Shaper: Lay your left hand on top of your right in front of you, palms together. Lift upward with your right arm while using your left arm to create resistance. Feel your right arm strengthening. Hold this flex for 5 seconds. Switch arms and repeat. Do twice on each side.

The Chest Firmer: Work your "pecs," or chest muscles, by putting your palms together in prayer position, then pressing your hands together for 5 seconds. Relax and repeat twice.

The Posture Perfecter: You can do this one while you're standing or sitting. Bend your elbows at a 90-degree angle, forearms parallel to the floor. Squeeze your shoulder blades down and together as you gently press your elbows back; this is a very subtle movement. Hold for 5 seconds, then release.

You now have more than one Fidget-cizer for every waking hour. But don't stop there! Be creative and find the movement that works for you—just remember to keep moving! Once Fidget-cize becomes a habit, you'll wonder how you ever sat still.

Remember: Food isn't our enemy; sitting still is!

14

Mind-Body-Spirit Routine

Our mind, our body and our spirit are inextricably connected. As we work together throughout these 28 days, I want you to remember this incredibly important connection. For a healthy body, you need to have a healthy mind and spirit. That's why my Mind-Body-Spirit Routine is such an integral part of this lose-the-last-10 plan.

These soothing moves can be done at any time of day—morning, noon or night. And they take only five minutes! I like to do them first thing in the morning—it's an invigorating, inspiring start to my day. If I'm on the road for business, I may do them at the end of a hard day—before I head off for a business dinner—to help me relax. Or you can do them right before bed to clear your mind, so you get a better night's sleep.

If you spend a lot of time sitting throughout the day, this routine is really for you. Hunching over a steering wheel or a computer keyboard can cause muscles and connective tissue to shorten, causing discomfort in your back. My Mind-Body-Spirit Routine can help unlock that tightness, almost like a natural massage.

Once you learn the moves, you'll be able to flow smoothly from one to the next to create a soothing sort of dance. Pay attention to your body as you hold the different poses. Maybe you'll notice that a particular area—your shoulders, your back or even your jaw—feels tense or tight. You can learn a lot about what's going on inside of your body, both physically and emotionally, by observing these subtle imbalances.

When you relax, you elongate your muscles, which can make you look up to five pounds thinner and an inch taller in just a few minutes! As you eliminate tension, your shoulders will relax and your back will lengthen. You'll carry yourself with more poise and grace. Best of all, you'll feel like a new person. Standing up and moving will be a freedom that you look forward to—not a chore.

Do one or two of these moves anytime you want to calm your nerves, soothe your spirit or work out the kinks. Or, if you want to feel totally revitalized, do the entire routine from start to finish. It will be five minutes well spent!

Stretches

Tai Chi Push and Pull
Stand with your feet hip-width apart, one leg in front of the other; your weight is over your back foot, hands in front of your chest, elbows bent out to the sides parallel to the floor, palms facing toward your heart. Shift your weight forward to your front foot as your hands push outward. For about 30 seconds, shift your weight backward and forward. This is a constant, flowing movement designed to get your "chi," or energy, flowing through your body. Switch legs and continue with the opposite leg in front.

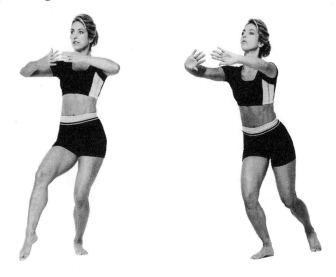

Reach-to-the-Sky Alignment Stretch

Stretch your way to a taller, leaner body, reverse the effects of slouching and unkink your back after you wake up with this arms-to-the-sky soother. With your legs together, stretch your arms over your head as if you're reaching for the clouds. Feel your spine elongate. Hold for 5 seconds. Relax for 2 seconds, then repeat.

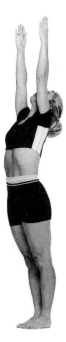

Height Enhancer

As you practice this move, feel the stretch through your waist. By lifting your rib cage and stretching the muscles along your spine, the Height Enhancer can make you look taller and leaner. Stand with your feet together and your knees slightly bent. With your arms extended straight up overhead, clasp your hands and stretch upward. Maintaining the stretch, bend your body to the right and hold for three deep breaths. Return to an upright position, then bend to the left. Hold for three deep breaths. Repeat.

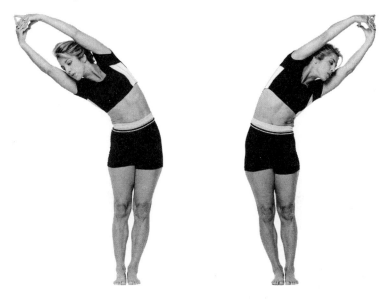

Yin and Yang Stretch

This is an excellent shoulder, neck and back stretch. Use it to lengthen your upper back and open up your chest to create a dancer's poise and grace. Stand with your feet a little wider than shoulder-width apart and your knees slightly bent. Place your hands above your knees to support your back. Keeping your back flat, rotate your torso to the right. Hold for 10 seconds. Return to center and repeat on the left side.

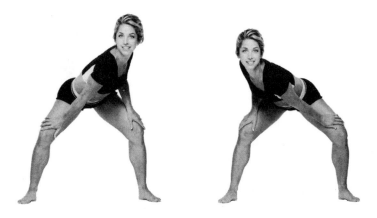

Soothing Back Stretch

Your spine is your lifeline! This is a wonderful way to wake up your spine, release tension in your back and get the blood circulating throughout your body. Stand with your feet shoulder-width apart, knees bent and arms relaxed. Tuck your chin to your chest and slowly roll down until your hands reach the floor. Your knees should be soft, not locked. Feel your upper body hang loosely forward from your hips. Hold for 10 seconds. Slowly roll up to an upright position one vertebra at a time. Repeat the entire move. The key to this stretch is to move *slowly*.

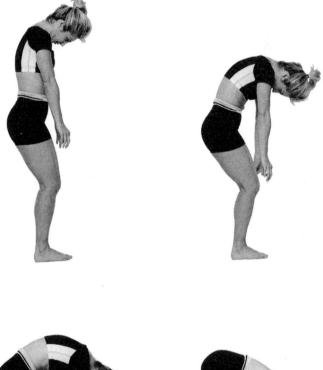

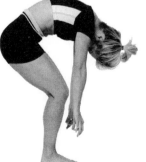

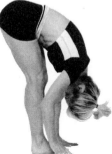

Part 4

Keeping It Off

15 | Beyond the First Four Weeks

Before we discuss how you can keep off the weight you've lost, I want you to take a few minutes to reflect on your recent accomplishments. Think about how light and limber your body feels. How lean and toned your muscles are. The new energy you have in your step. The smile on your face. As you look both inside yourself and in the mirror, you see a brand-new, healthier you. Feels wonderful, doesn't it?

By now, you've figured out the secret to maintaining your ideal weight and feeling great: *balance*. You can't eat just one huge meal or exercise just one day a week. To remain healthy, you need to achieve balance in every aspect of your life—your eating habits, your workouts, your job and your relationships. Think of your life as a car with four wheels: If one of the wheels is flat, forget about driving!

The road ahead will have many ups and downs, and it's easy to lose control. Your challenge from now on will be to maintain the balance that you've established during the last four weeks. You don't just wake up one day and have a guaranteed harmonious life. As in learning to play a sport or a musical instrument, you need to practice—and keep practicing and practicing and practicing.

For the past 28 days, you've had set meal and exercise plans to guide you. But I've also given you the knowledge to go out and do it on your own. This book is full of tips for losing the last 10 pounds, and the same tips apply to maintaining weight loss. Use every one of them. Keep a copy of your daily checklist on your refrigerator, on your nightstand or in your personal organizer. Continue keeping tabs on your food intake and workouts by logging them in a journal.

This healthy and doable plan is designed to be a blueprint for the rest of your life. As long as you continue working out, you can increase your caloric intake by up to 2,000 a day—but those calories should come from nutrient-dense foods, not junk. Of course, it's OK to treat yourself once in a while, provided that you get back on track right away. Whatever happens, don't even consider cutting back on exercise—it's the missing link for anyone trying to lose or maintain his or her weight.

Just because the program is over doesn't mean you need to put this book aside. In Chapter 18, you'll find 28 new healthy, delicious recipes to try. Or take your favorite dishes from the last 28 days and incorporate them into your weekly meal plans. You can continue to do your weekly aerobic and toning workouts; just be sure to keep changing your routine so your muscles stay challenged.

Life is full of holidays, festivities and temptations, and I don't want you to miss out! If you step off course, don't worry—you can always get back on track. No matter what, don't let discouragement or disappointment serve as an excuse to abandon your healthy habits. You'll only be defeating yourself. Your best defense is a good offense—and the best offense is a strong, nimble body!

One of the most effective ways to stay on course is to be a proactive problem solver! People who successfully lose weight and keep it off learn to identify their specific obstacles and overcome them. Try to pinpoint likely pitfalls and map out a plan of action that addresses them. Let's say you constantly fall prey to the hoard of junk food that you purchase for your kids. A possible solution might be to store the junk and the good-for-you snacks in separate cabinets—one for them and one for you. This will establish boundaries that prevent you from being tempted. With a little ingenuity, you can overcome any problem.

Another key to continuing success is to stay organized. Planning ahead can prevent last-minute phone calls for fattening pizza or Chinese take-out. If you're cooking for one or two, double up and freeze half. On Sundays, I plan all my meals for the week and purchase my groceries. Then I cook a big roasted chicken, low-fat turkey chili or a vegetable lasagna; we eat some for dinner and freeze the leftovers to use later in the week. This way, my kitchen work is cut in half, allowing more precious minutes for other activities and exercise (and leaving fewer dirty pots and pans). That's my idea of a relaxing evening!

Now that you've succeeded in reaching your goal weight, you'll need to dangle a new carrot in front of your eyes to stay motivated. Train for a 5K race. Plan an active vacation—a skiing, cycling or hiking trip. Or make yourself a bet: Seal $100 in an envelope to be put toward a brand-new outfit if you haven't gained weight in six months. Talk about a reason to move!

A fourth, highly effective—and fun—way to keep on track is to make good health a group effort. Research shows that a good support system is crucial to long-term weight loss. Family and friends can't read your mind, so reach out to them and let them in on your goals. If you're juggling household duties and kids, ask a friend to baby-sit or recruit your spouse to help with the dishes while you aerobicize. Asking for help isn't a sign of weakness or incompetance—it's a sign of intelligence.

Most important, even though you may be busy taking care of others, don't think of caring for yourself as a luxury—it's a necessity! Staying fit and healthy will make you a better caretaker. It's one of the best things that you can do for the people you love. You'll have more energy and more patience, and you'll be more fun to be around.

Strive for balance—it's what we all need to be truly happy. A healthy body and a healthy mind will help you keep those last 10 pounds off—forever!

16

What Works for Me

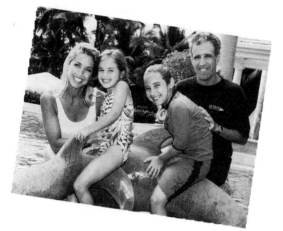

Me, Jeff, and our beautiful girls, Katie and Kelly, on a break taping my TV show Fit and Lite.

People are always asking me what my life is really like, how I make time for exercise and what I eat. They're usually surprised by my answers: I have a fulfilling family life, I don't spend all day working out and I'm a sucker for cookies! I certainly don't want to discourage you or lead you to believe that I'm some sort of genetic anomaly. Just the opposite: I want you to realize that a fit, toned body is 100 percent attainable for practically everyone.

On the following pages, I'm going to walk you through a typical day in the Austin household. You'll see how I manage to sneak in exercise despite a schedule that includes two kids, home-cooked meals and a full-time job. It isn't always easy—and sometimes we find ourselves eating TV dinners instead of fresh spinach salad. But even on days that I don't have time for a full 30-minute workout, I'm getting exercise. Bottom line: If you want to keep those 10 pounds off, you *must* move—working your muscles is the only way to keep your metabolism revved! To see what I mean, read on.

6:30 A.M. I rise and shine with a smile, then take three deep breaths for oxygen power. Part of me wants to crawl back under the covers, but I know that five minutes of Tai Chi, QiGong and yoga will get my blood flowing and wake up my entire body.

Before starting, I down two full cups of water—I haven't had any for at least eight hours, and my muscles will need it to perform.

6:45 A.M. Since I did a toning routine yesterday, I switch to a calorie-blasting aerobic workout for the next 30 minutes. I lace up my shoes and head out for a run along the Potomac (on other days, I do my TV show on Lifetime). I always try to do my workout in the morning to make sure some "emergency" doesn't circumvent it later on—and so I won't have to worry about it all day long. Just thinking about my "splurge" last night makes me pick up the pace!

7:15 A.M. Wow! That was work. To prevent stiff muscles, I stretch my buttocks, thighs and calves. Takes an extra five minutes but pays in the end. No pun intended.

7:20 A.M. I wake up the kids, then run upstairs—three flights total!—to shower and dress. I've learned to streamline my routine so it takes only 20 minutes to get ready.

7:40 A.M. Back downstairs to prepare a healthy sit-down breakfast for Jeff, Katie, Kelly and me. First, a big glass of water and Florida grapefruit juice. We all love cereal, especially with add-ons like berries, bananas and peaches. Yogurt, skim milk or soy milk on top adds protein as well.

8:00 A.M. Time to Fidget-cize! I do a buns firmer while brushing my teeth (see page 204).

8:05 A.M. Prepare lunch (turkey or tuna sandwiches) and snacks (apples, carrot sticks and oatmeal cookies) for the kids and me. Fill up five bottles of water for the day (I use sports bottles as well as empty Evian bottles that I've washed with hot, soapy water), then drive the children to school. As a mom, I'm always running around in the car, taking or picking up one or both of my girls for their activities, so I store a bottle in the front seat.

8:30 A.M. Stuck in traffic on the way back to work. No road rage—frowns cause wrinkles. While waiting, I do 15 tummy tucks—holding for 4 seconds and releasing for 4 seconds.

9:00 A.M. Arrive at my office (in my home) and immediately get on the phone—my days are always filled with lots of calls! Do 30 triceps toners while talking—15 with each arm. I have a heavy paperweight to hold for resistance. Plus, I always try to walk or pace while I'm talking. Remember: Standing—or better yet, walking—burns more calories than sitting!

10:00 A.M. Fidget-cize No. 3—a supported back stretch (see page 211). Send a fax after pulling those kinks out.

10:30 A.M. Energy lift time. Snack on my favorite sweet potato pick-me-up (see recipe, page 254). Then it's back to the job. . . .

11:00 A.M. Time for more fidgeting! This time, I do wall sits (page 207) while talking on the phone.

12:00 P.M. I can't wait to get out of a chair and into fresh air. Before lunch, I take a brisk 10-minute walk outdoors. It's a beautiful day, so I eat my turkey, spinach and tomato sandwich as I amble along the river. To satisfy a postlunch chocolate craving, I nibble on a Sweet 'N Low Chocolate Wafer candy—low fat and sugar free. Yum!

1:00 P.M. Back to work. Hunching over a computer is tiring, so I remind myself to straighten up. Good posture makes you look thinner and can help prevent backaches!

2:00 P.M. Flip through the newspaper to see what's happening in the world. Grab a dumbbell and do seated biceps curls (two 12-rep sets with each arm) while I read up on the latest health news.

3:00 P.M. Time to pick up the kids from school. It's also time for Fidget-cize, so I do a waist twist while waiting in the car-pool line.

3:30 P.M. Everyone's hungry when we get home, so I pour three glasses of skim milk and hand out ginger snaps.

4:00 P.M. While the girls do their homework, I do a quick telephone interview. When I hang up, I practice a few of my kickboxing moves—front kick, side kick, left jab, right hook—to get the oxygen flowing again.

5:00 P.M. Every day after work, I try to go outside with Katie and Kelly for at least 20 minutes for fresh air and exercise. Today we play catch with a big rubber ball. I can't count how many lunges I do picking up wild throws. Great for the thighs! Next, we take Madonna, our tireless dog, for a walk.

6:00 P.M. I fire up the grill, then do Saddlebag Slimmers (page 206) while preparing salad for dinner.

6:30 P.M. Sit down for a relaxing meal with my family. Everyone loves grilled chicken and roasted potato wedges balanced with spinach, carrot and tomato salad (even the girls!). Dessert is fresh melon and blueberries topped with vanilla yogurt (Katie and Kelly get two scoops of ice cream).

7:00 P.M. Jeff helps me clean up after dinner (he's always a good sport!); I do arabesques at the kitchen sink while I rinse dishes. Then we all hang out as a family—watching TV, playing a board game or, on some nights, going to Kelly's baseball and basketball practices. I cherish the time that we spend as a foursome.

8:00 P.M. Hang up the invisible "Kitchen Is Closed" sign. We put the girls to bed with a good story or a chat about their day. Then Jeff and I watch a little TV, talk and relax together. Even though he laughs, I do push-ups and crunches during commercials.

9:00 P.M. I take a few minutes to review my day—not just listing things to be done, but reflecting on my accomplishments, too. I like to remind myself of all the positives in my life—the counting blessings bit that we discussed in Week 4—and think of how I can pass the secrets of contentment along to you. Above all, I remind myself that LIFE IS AN ADVENTURE! And I thank God for another great day.

10:00 P.M. We head for bed. A busy body needs time to regroup, so I always try to get *at least* eight hours of sleep each night. One last exercise—I set the alarm.

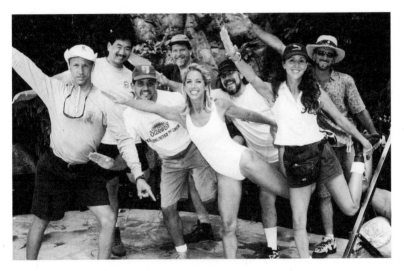

Me and my crew for my TV show, shooting on location in Hawaii.

17

Ask Denise!

Many people stop me in airports and at personal appearances to ask questions about losing weight and getting in shape. In this chapter, I've included answers to 20 of your top questions. As you make the transition from weight loss to weight maintenance, use this information to prevent a relapse and to help you continue making progress. Remember: Knowledge is power!

Q. How can I find time for meaningful exercise?
A. You need to *make* time. There's one main difference between people who exercise regularly and those who don't: Regular exercisers make their workouts a priority. If you've got a busy schedule, you may want to exercise first thing in the morning. The blow-off potential only grows as the clock ticks and you become engrossed in the day's activities. Try to streamline your life as much as possible. Don't overbook yourself. Learn to set boundaries. And be flexible. If you can't spare a whole hour, use five or 10 minutes to isolate and strengthen a muscle. Target exercises are great for toning—and you don't need to be in fitness clothes to do them. Or turn your commute into a workout. A brisk 10- to 20-minute walk to the office or train station will do nicely in a pinch. Shorten your lunch hour and walk for 20 minutes. At

home you can use the stairs for aerobic climbs or turn on some music with a beat and dance away. If you find 10 minutes here and there, you just might end up with the required 30 minutes of exercise before you know it!

Q. Won't I get hungrier when I exercise?
A. Yes and no. Research shows that a premeal workout (even if it's just a 10-minute walk) can help suppress your appetite, so you're less likely to overindulge when you sit down to eat. But since exercise speeds up your metabolism, you're burning more calories throughout the day—so you may feel hungrier in general. Fortunately, since you're working it off, you can afford to eat a little more—as long as you're trying to maintain, not lose, weight. I'm not giving you the green light to overeat, I'm merely pointing out the need to keep your body well-fueled with good-for-you foods. If you're trying to lose weight, drinking lots of water will help fill you up and keep your stomach from growling.

Q. After I have lost the 10 pounds, what do I eat?
A. First of all, don't even think of returning to the bad habits that got you trying to lose weight in the first place—like skipping breakfast, skimping on fruits and vegetables or surviving on junk food. Stay with my general plan of healthful small meals and modest snacks, increasing the calorie count gradually up to about 2,000 a day. Have fun developing new recipes based on the ingredients in my meal plans.

Q. How can I drink two or three quarts of water a day?
A. Plan ahead. You can buy bottled water by the carload or spend a few minutes filling up empty bottles in the morning like I do. Next, space it out. Have a big glass of water before breakfast, mid-morning, just before and after lunch. Half done! Drink up in the midafternoon, before and after dinner, and midevening. No problem! Finally, take advantage of every water fountain that you pass.

Q. When you talk about stretching, do you simply mean making your muscles feel better after exercise?
A. Yes, but it's about much, much more. Stretching is certainly a feel-good action—it comforts your body and releases tension, but it also conditions your muscles for moving. The more flexible you are, the less likely you are to get injured (and you know what an injury can do to your waistline!). Stretches also help work out the kinks in your neck, back, arm and leg muscles to improve your posture and even make you look taller.

Q. Should I throw away my "fat" clothes?
A. If you have to ask that question, then you aren't ready to believe in yourself—and less likely to keep off the weight. Don't think failure. And don't even worry about your closet until you first think only of health, happiness and pride in your new strength.

Q. How fast should I walk for good aerobic exercise?
A. An average speed for beginners is 3 to 3.5 miles per hour, or 1 mile in 18 to 20 minutes. You don't need a fancy pedometer—just map out a few half-mile and one-mile routes in your car and time yourself. For starters, a good goal would be walking 2 to 3 miles four or five times a week.

Q. Even when I lose weight, I don't like the way my hips and rear end look. Can I reduce a specific area?
A. Unfortunately, it's true that "spot reducing," or losing fat from one specific area, is impossible. You'd have to lose fat from all over your body, and even then there's no guarantee that you'll lose it from your hips and buttocks. But you *can* improve the look of those areas by doing toning exercises. The moves on pages 179 to 193 of this book can help. Don't expect a miracle, but if you keep at it, you can change your shape for the better in just four to six weeks.

Q. How can I avoid gaining weight over the holidays?
A. Remember the basic rules. Avoid fat-filled, non-nutritious nibbles. Drink lots of water or seltzer instead of alcoholic beverages. Have a healthy fiber-filled snack—an apple, an orange or a bowl of whole-grain cereal—to decrease your appetite before hitting your aunt Martha's buffet or your company's Christmas fete. At parties, fill your plate with veggies and a bit of dip. Order fish in restaurants and seek out fruit or sorbet if everyone is insisting on dessert. And pass on coffee if you can't drink it without lots of sugar and cream.

Q. On nights that I don't have time to cook, can I substitute a frozen dinner?
A. Packaged foods tend to be loaded with sodium, but if you don't have time to prepare your own meal, a frozen dinner is certainly better than stopping at McDonald's or some other fast-food restaurant. Since frozen dinners tend to be low on vegetables, fix yourself a small spinach salad or steam some fresh or frozen veggies to add to your meal.

Q. How can I get rid of my cellulite?
A. I get this question all the time, and unfortunately, there is no easy

solution. Cellulite is essentially subcutaneous fat in the buns and thighs that most women experience in varying degrees—myself included. This fat is no different from fat in any other part of your body, except that it can be a little harder to lose. The key is to reduce your overall body fat by engaging in regular aerobic exercise and eating a sensible, low-fat diet. As I mentioned earlier, toning exercises can also help give this area a smoother, firmer look.

Q. How often should I change my workout routine?
A. As often as possible. There's some evidence that your body starts to adjust to a workout after about three months, but I personally believe that you should change your program more frequently. Over time, your muscles adjust to an exercise routine, essentially "memorizing" your workout. They stop working as hard, and you stop seeing results. Variety is also key to preventing boredom and overuse injuries. While I follow the same basic cardio, strength and flexibility program every week, I try to throw in new exercises or vary my intensity with each workout. Do your best!

Q. I do crunches religiously, but I don't seem to get more toned in my abdominal region. What's my problem?
A. You may need to spend *less* time doing crunches and *more* time on the treadmill, stair climber or stationary bike. Contrary to popular belief, abdominal tone doesn't come from doing a million crunches. In fact, you may already have abs of steel—they simply may be covered by a layer of insulation. So instead of doing 10 or 15 minutes of crunches, try doing 3 to 5 minutes of exercises targeting different abdominal muscles as well as your lower back; focus on using good form and really tightening those muscles. Then spend the extra 5 to 7 minutes burning fat with a cardio activity such as running or cycling.

Q. How many fat grams should I eat per day?
A. It depends on how many calories you're consuming. I aim to get about 20 to 25 percent of my daily calories from fat—and since I eat about 2,000 calories every day, that's about 44 to 55 grams. Even more important than the total number of fat grams: how much *saturated fat* you're taking in. Saturated fat is the kind that damages your arteries, putting you at higher risk of heart attack. No more than 10 percent of your daily calories should come from saturated fat; for a 2,000-calorie-per-day diet, that means about 22 grams or less.

Q. I know a lot of people who have lost weight by cutting out carbohydrates. Is this a good way to trim down?

A. Absolutely not. Carbohydrates provide instant energy, so you need them to fuel your workouts and all your daily activities. In fact, high-carb diets are the only proven way to lose weight and keep it off; they're also associated with longer life spans. While it isn't a bad idea to cut back on simple carbohydrates, such as white bread, crackers and frozen yogurt—these foods tend to be low in nutrients and high in sugar—complex carbs like potatoes, oatmeal and whole-grain bread provide essential nutrients and fiber. The key is to choose your carbs wisely; never attempt to eliminate entire food groups—an unhealthy move that will set you up for failure.

Q. What percentage of body fat should I aim for?
A. The average body-fat recommendation for women is 22 to 24 percent. But every woman and physique is different, so I recommend that you remain where you feel and look your best. Some women look better with a little extra fat; others need to carry less. Being healthy is most important!

Q. Shouldn't I lose weight before I start to lift weights?
A. No. This is a common misconception. A lot of people think that if they have fat on their body and they start to lift weights, their fat will turn into muscle. This is impossible. Fat is fat and muscle is muscle! In fact, lifting weights actually contributes to fat loss, since the added muscle increases your metabolism. And speeding up that metabolism helps you to lose weight even more quickly.

Q. I have a bad back. What are my best workout options?
A. Strengthening the muscles surrounding your spine is vital for a healthy back, so I suggest a regular program of abdominal and lower-back exercises. Keeping your hamstrings strong and flexible can also help prevent back pain. Yoga is an excellent workout for all of the above. Swimming and walking are other great aerobic activities that don't put a lot of stress on your spine. Of course, if you're experiencing severe back pain, consult your doctor before engaging in any form of exercise.

Q. If I'm going to do toning and cardio on the same day, which should I do first?
A. It really depends on what your goal is. If you're focused on shaping and defining your muscles, do the toning moves first, so you feel fresh and full of energy. If you're trying to build up your aerobic endurance or train for an event, like a 10K walk or weekend bike trip, you may want to do cardio first. Personally, I like

to start with cardio; it helps warm up my muscles and gets me pumped for my toning workout. But decide for yourself!

Q. I've heard that stair running or walking is a great workout. Do you recommend it?

A. Definitely. People all over the country are doing stair workouts to burn fat and build muscle. It's terrific for the buns, thighs and calves. And if you run or walk quickly, you work your heart anaerobically—a fabulous way to really blast flab and improve cardio conditioning. You can use the staircase in your home; better yet, find three or four consecutive flights in a nearby park or building. Vary your workout by climbing two or three stairs at a time or walking up and down sideways (facing the banister). Or, if you have a solid fitness base, try walking a flight, then jogging or sprinting up a flight; continue alternating walking and sprinting throughout your workout. One caveat: No matter what, always walk down the stairs—never run. Running will put far too much pressure on your knees, and you could lose your footing and fall. Don't risk it!

18 | Extra Recipes

As promised, here are more recipes for you to substitute into the 28 daily meal plans or use after the four weeks are done. They're some of my favorites—and my family's favorites, too. Most of the recipes can be prepared in 30 minutes or less. As a busy mom, I know how important "quick and easy" is. All of them include lots of fresh, nutrient-dense foods. While a few of the dinners may sound a bit exotic, all of the ingredients can be purchased in the supermarket— no special trips to specialty food stores required. They're designed to serve four to six people. If you're cooking for one, simply cut the recipes down—or save the extra to eat later in the week. Enjoy!

Breakfasts

SUPERCHARGED BREAKFAST IN A BOWL

This all-in-one breakfast packs in lots of essential vitamins, minerals, protein and fiber. I eat this on days that I film my TV show. It's sweet, crunchy and satisfying! Serves 4

    2 medium red Florida grapefruits, peeled, cut crosswise in
        half and separated into sections

1 cup sliced strawberries, raspberries or blueberries
2 small bananas, sliced
2 tablespoons honey combined with ½ teaspoon cinnamon
    (optional)
½ cup low-fat granola cereal (optional)
1 cup strawberry, raspberry or vanilla nonfat yogurt

Divide fruit between four cereal bowls. Drizzle with honey mixture, if desired. Top with granola, if desired, and yogurt.

CALORIES	243
FAT	1 GRAM
CALCIUM	28 MG
FIBER	9 GRAMS

FRUIT SMOOTHIE

Another great way to start the day, or to give you a boost of energy whenever you need it!   Serves 4

3 8-ounce containers low-fat yogurt, fruit flavored
4 5-inch bananas
2 cups frozen strawberries
16 ounces orange juice
16 ounces nonfat milk

Blend together the above ingredients until smooth. (I use my Osterizer blender.) Pour into four tall glasses and serve cold.

CALORIES	320
FAT	1 GRAM
CALCIUM	60 MG
FIBER	4.5 GRAMS

Salads

FRESH SPINACH AND GRAPEFRUIT SALAD

This fiber- and calcium-rich salad blends several distinct tastes and textures. Every bite will be a delightful surprise!   Serves 4

1 10-ounce package washed spinach leaves, stemmed
    and torn
2 medium red Florida grapefruits, peeled, cut crosswise in
    half and separated into sections

1 red bell pepper, cut into short, thin strips
½ cup sliced green onions
½ cup light honey Dijon or Italian salad dressing
¼ cup low-fat bacon bits (optional)
¼ cup fat-free seasoned croutons

In a large bowl, combine spinach, grapefruit sections, bell pepper and green onions. Add dressing and toss well. Transfer mixture to four serving plates. Sprinkle with bacon bits and croutons.

CALORIES	147
FAT	3 GRAMS
CALCIUM	100 MG
FIBER	9 GRAMS

For a variation on this terrific salad, throw in a little chicken, as follows:

Brush four 4-ounce skinless and boneless chicken breasts with 2 additional tablespoons of salad dressing. Grill over medium coals or broil 4 to 5 inches from the heat source for 5 minutes per side, or until chicken is cooked through. Cut grilled chicken crosswise into ½-inch-thick pieces and arrange over spinach and grapefruit salad prepared as recipe directs.

CALORIES	282
FAT	7 GRAMS
CALCIUM	111 MG
FIBER	9 GRAMS

TUNA AND WHITE BEAN SALAD

An elegant lunch that's easy and low-calorie. I love to use sweet Vidalia onions, and, as a garnish, cherry tomatoes and black olives.　　　　　　　　　　　　　　　　　　　　　　　Serves 4

1 6½-ounce can water-packed tuna, drained
1 14-ounce can white beans, drained
3 tablespoons onion, chopped
½ pound green beans, steamed and patted dry
4 tablespoons fresh basil, chopped
Juice of 1 lemon
1 teaspoon Dijon mustard
2 teaspoons red wine vinegar
1 garlic clove, finely minced

2 tablespoons olive oil
4 cups Bibb or romaine lettuce leaves

Place tuna in a mixing bowl, breaking up chunks with a fork. Toss tuna with white beans, onion, green beans and basil. Squeeze lemon juice over mixture and toss lightly. In a separate bowl combine mustard, vinegar and garlic. Stir briskly to mix. Add olive oil in a slow, steady, thin stream. Continue stirring until smooth. Pour dressing over tuna mixture and toss. Serve over lettuce leaves. This salad may be served cold or at room temperature.

CALORIES   208
FAT   6 GRAMS
CALCIUM   12 MG
FIBER   9.1 GRAMS

AUSTIN LENTIL AND AVOCADO SALAD

Sometimes I serve this as a healthy dip with low-fat, baked tortilla chips.   Serves 4

1 cup lentils
½ cup low-fat sour cream
Juice of 1 lime or lemon
1 tablespoon cilantro, chopped
1 tomato, chopped
Salt and pepper, to taste
½ cup canned black beans
1 ripe avocado, peeled, pitted and cubed
4 cups endive or Bibb lettuce leaves

Cook lentils according to package in water or broth. Drain. In a bowl, whisk together sour cream, lime or lemon juice, cilantro, tomato and salt and pepper. Add beans and lentils, and stir. Add avocado and spoon over lettuce leaves. *Note: Don't add the avocado until you are ready to serve the salad or it will turn brown.*

CALORIES   253
FAT   8 GRAMS
CALCIUM   11 MG
FIBER   12.1 GRAMS

WARM CHICKEN SALAD WITH ORANGES

The oranges give this salad a light, citrus flavor, not to mention a vitamin C boost! This is also one of the quickest meals in my recipe file.   Serves 4

1/2 pound fresh snow peas
2 chicken breasts, boneless and skinless
1/4 cup flour (to coat)
1 tablespoon vegetable oil
4 cups salad greens
2 fresh seedless Florida oranges, peeled and sectioned
1/4 cup scallions, sliced
1 tablespoon lime juice
1 tablespoon orange juice
1/2 cup seedless green grapes, halved
2 teaspoons Dijon mustard
1 tablespoon olive oil

Place snow peas in a pot of boiling water. Blanch for 2 minutes, then plunge peas into a bowl of ice water to stop the cooking process. Drain and set aside. Pound chicken breasts on cooking board with the back of your hand and coat lightly with flour. Heat vegetable oil in skillet and add chicken, cooking about 4 minutes per side until nicely browned. Arrange salad greens on four plates. Slice chicken breasts into thin strips and place on greens. Add snow peas and arrange nicely. To the warm skillet, add orange sections, scallions, lime juice, orange juice, grapes and mustard. Simmer over low heat for several minutes. Stir in olive oil and blend over low heat for a few seconds with a spoon. Ladle orange sauce over chicken and snow peas.

CALORIES	239
FAT	9 GRAMS
CALCIUM	9 MG
FIBER	5.6 GRAMS

Dinners

SAVORY CHICKEN SAUTÉ

Here's another nice citrusy twist to chicken—one of my family's favorite sources of lean protein.   Serves 4

2 cups brown rice, quick cooking
2 cups assorted cut salad bar vegetables (broccoli florets, shredded carrots, diced bell peppers and diced zucchini or yellow squash)
4 4-ounce chicken breast halves, skinless and boneless
1 teaspoon dried rosemary, crushed
½ teaspoon salt
¼ teaspoon freshly ground black pepper
1 tablespoon olive oil
½ cup chopped onion
2 cloves garlic, minced
½ cup canned chicken broth, low sodium
1 tablespoon cornstarch
¼ cup orange marmalade
2 medium red Florida grapefruits, peeled and cut crosswise in half, and separated into sections.

Prepare rice according to package. Stir in vegetables during last 5 minutes of cooking. While rice is cooking, sprinkle chicken with rosemary, salt and pepper. Heat oil in large skillet over medium heat. Add chicken, onion and garlic; cook for 5 minutes. Turn chicken, stir onion and garlic and cook for an additional 5 minutes or until chicken is cooked through. Transfer chicken to a plate and set aside. Combine chicken broth and cornstarch, mixing well. Add to skillet; cook and stir until sauce thickens. Stir in marmalade, add grapefruit and mix well. Return chicken to skillet. Turn to coat with sauce.

Transfer rice and vegetable mixture to four serving plates. Spoon chicken, grapefruit and sauce mixture over rice.

CALORIES	493
FAT	9 GRAMS
CALCIUM	63 MG
FIBER	10 GRAMS

JEFF'S FAVORITE BURGERS

My husband is a grill master! He discovered that mixing meats helps us reduce fat and calories while giving us the juiciest and most flavorful burgers on the block. Serves 4

2 tomatoes, peeled, seeded and chopped
1 avocado, peeled and chopped
1/4 cup nonfat or low-fat sour cream
1 tablespoon cilantro, minced
1/2 pound lean ground turkey
1/2 pound lean ground beef or lamb
1/4 cup medium-hot salsa
1 teaspoon chili powder
1/4 teaspoon ground cumin
4 hamburger rolls, preferably whole wheat
Lettuce leaves and tomato slices for garnish

Stir together tomatoes, avocado, sour cream and cilantro. Set aside. In a mixing bowl, combine meats, salsa, chili powder and ground cumin. Blend well, using your hands, and form into four patties. On a well-oiled grill, cook burgers until done. We usually grill them for about 5 minutes on each side. Assemble the burgers by placing a roll on each plate, top the rolls with tomato and avocado mixture, place hamburger on next and garnish with lettuce leaves and tomato slices. Enjoy!

CALORIES	374
FAT	25 GRAMS
CALCIUM	4 MG
FIBER	3 GRAMS

PORTOBELLO PASTA

My vegetarian pasta includes a lot of garlicky veggies and very thin spaghetti or cappelini. The large Portobello mushrooms have become a staple and are considered the "steak" version of a mushroom. Many supermarkets now carry them presliced. Of course, they are very low in calories with no cholesterol. Serves 4

4 large Portobello mushrooms
2 small zucchini, cut into 1/4-inch lengthwise slices
Olive oil, for brushing
12 ounces thin spaghetti, cooked al dente and drained
2 tablespoons olive oil

3 cloves garlic, minced
2 large plum tomatoes, diced
Salt and freshly ground pepper, to taste
½ cup fresh basil leaves, shredded

Brush each side of mushrooms and zucchini slices with olive oil. Heat grill to medium-high. When hot, grill mushrooms until brown on each side. Grill zucchini slices quickly on one side only. Slice mushrooms. Reserve. Prepare pasta. Heat olive oil in a large saucepan over medium-high heat. When hot, add garlic and plum tomatoes and sauté 1 minute. Add salt and freshly ground pepper to taste. Toss for a few minutes to heat all. Place on individual serving plates and top with shredded basil.

CALORIES	268
FAT	11 GRAMS
CALCIUM	4 MG
FIBER	3.5 GRAMS

JEFF'S SPICY SHRIMP ADOBO

An adobo is basically a marinade, Latin-style. This combination of spices and herbs adds character without heaviness. It can be a dry spice blend or wet, like this one. Make large batches of this basic adobo since it's a good, all-purpose marinade. Shrimp or chicken need only about 2 to 8 hours to marinate. Pork or beef can marinate overnight.   Serves 4

FRESH CILANTRO ADOBO

1½ cups fresh cilantro (leaves and stems)
2 teaspoons ground cumin
2 teaspoons dried oregano
2 teaspoons dried thyme
2 teaspoons pepper
1 tablespoon salt
½ cup white onion, coarsely chopped
4 cloves garlic, coarsely chopped
1 cup white wine vinegar
½ cup vegetable oil

1 pound large shrimp, peeled and deveined
2 cups cooked rice
1 tomato, sliced

Place all of the adobo ingredients, except vegetable oil, in a blender or food processor. Puree on high speed. Drizzle in vegetable oil. Marinate shrimp in about 1 cup of adobo for 2 to 8 hours in the refrigerator. (Save the rest of the marinade in the refrigerator.) Heat a large nonstick sauté pan over high heat. When hot, add shrimp in a single layer and sear until pink on each side. Do not overcook. Divide rice and tomato slices between four plates. Serve shrimp over rice and tomato slices.

CALORIES	220
FAT	11 GRAMS
CALCIUM	2 MG
FIBER	0.3 GRAM

GREEK STUFFED BELL PEPPERS

Simply scrumptious, these stuffed bells are inspired by the Cyclades island of Santorini, where food is uncomplicated and all the fresh indigenous ingredients are put to use. I love it because it's a whole meal in a "shell."   Serves 4

4 red or yellow bell peppers
2 cups fat-free ricotta
2 cloves garlic, minced
1/3 cup feta cheese, crumbled
1 egg white, lightly beaten
2 teaspoons oregano leaves
1/4 cup walnuts, chopped and toasted
3/4 cup fresh bread crumbs
2 teaspoons olive oil

Place peppers in a large Pyrex pie plate, cover with plastic wrap and microwave for 4 to 6 minutes on 100 percent power, rotating after 2 minutes. Peppers should soften, but not collapse. Cut off tops and remove seeds. Leave peppers in the plate with the lids on the side. Preheat the broiler. In a small bowl, combine ricotta, garlic, feta, egg, oregano, and walnuts. Fill each pepper with this mixture. Mix bread crumbs with olive oil and sprinkle over cheese filling. Cover the stuffed peppers loosely with the plastic wrap and microwave again for 8 to 12 minutes, rotating after 4 minutes. The filling should be hot in the center. Remove the plastic wrap and broil the peppers for a minute or two to brown the crumbs. Serve immediately, allowing one stuffed pepper per person.

CALORIES	346
FAT	11 GRAMS

CALCIUM   2 MG
FIBER   0.3 GRAM

DENISE'S ISLAND SWEET POTATO CHOWDER

When icy winter winds blow from the north, I like to transport myself to a southern sun-drenched island with this amazingly carefree recipe. With the help of some quality canned products, you can prepare this chowder in about 10 minutes.   Serves 4

    1 16-ounce can sweet potatoes or yams, drained
    2½ cups vegetable or chicken stock
    1 cup 2% milk
    1-pound bag frozen broccoli, corn and red bell peppers
    1 15½-ounce can black beans, rinsed and drained
    1 teaspoon oregano
    ½ cup chopped scallions
    Hot sauce (optional)

In a blender or food processor, puree sweet potatoes, stock and milk. Place sweet potato puree in a medium saucepan and heat over medium-high heat. When hot, add remaining ingredients and stir until all are hot. Serve immediately.

CALORIES   377
FAT   5 GRAMS
CALCIUM   18 MG
FIBER   17.7 GRAMS

TILAPIA WITH BALSAMIC GLAZE

Low-fat, fast and multipurpose, this glazed sauce can be used on almost any variety of grilled, broiled, baked or sautéed fish, or even on chicken. Make the most of the farmer's market by serving an abundance of produce, such as broccoli and corn on the cob, with the fish.   Serves 4

    1 tablespoon olive oil
    2 tablespoons shallots, minced
    2 cloves fresh garlic, minced
    1 tablespoon lemon juice
    Zest from 1 lemon
    2 tablespoons balsamic vinegar
    ¼ cup dry vermouth
    ½ cup clam juice or vegetable broth

2 tablespoons fresh basil, chopped
4 6-ounce tilapia fillets, or any mild white fish
Salt and fresh ground pepper to taste

In a medium saucepan, heat olive oil over medium-high heat. Add shallots and garlic and cook for 2 minutes. Add remaining ingredients except basil and fish. Bring to a boil and cook for 5 minutes until liquid has reduced a bit. Set aside until fish is grilled. Turn on grill to high heat. Salt and pepper fish. For ½-inch-thick fillets, grill 2 to 4 minutes per side, depending on thickness of fillet. Stir basil into the glaze and spoon over fish fillets. Serve at once.

CALORIES	189
FAT	5 GRAMS
CALCIUM	4 MG
FIBER	0.1 GRAM

KELLY'S CLEVER GAZPACHO

You'll find this complete meal perfect for a holiday out of town or as a quick fix at the beach. Even the girls love it, especially Kelly! The no-cook chilled gazpacho is virtually prep and appliance-free, but tastes fresh and homemade. Serve some crunchy bagel chips on the side. Serves 4

2 cups (16 ounces) salsa (I use mild)
Juice of 1 lime
1½ cups cucumber, diced
½ cup scallions, diced
2 16-ounce cans cannelini or navy beans, rinsed and drained
1½ to 2 cups V-8 juice

In a large bowl, place salsa, lime juice, cucumber, scallions and beans. Pour in enough V-8 juice to make a chunky, slightly thick soup. A few ice cubes can be stirred in until melted to chill soup if ingredients were not previously chilled. Serve immediately or refrigerate to allow flavors to blend.

CALORIES	220
FAT	1 GRAM
CALCIUM	8 MG
FIBER	20.9 GRAMS

MEDITERRANEAN RELISH ON POLENTA ROUNDS

Have you tried polenta in trendy restaurants? Now you can make that delicious corn-based dish easily at home! Polenta is now available in ready-to-go tubes. It's fat-free and quite good. Just grill or brown the slices and top with something exotic—like this Mediterranean relish!   Serves 4

1 eggplant (about 12 ounces), sliced into ½-inch-thick rounds
Olive oil for brushing and drizzling
3 cloves garlic, peeled
Salt and freshly ground pepper, to taste
1 tablespoon salt-packed or canned capers, well rinsed
    and drained
2 anchovy fillets, well rinsed and drained (optional)
½ teaspoon fresh thyme leaves, minced
1 tablespoon dark rum or brandy (optional)
2 plum tomatoes, diced
⅔ cup jarred roasted red bell pepper, diced
2 tablespoons flat-leaf parsley, freshly chopped
Salt, to taste
1 tube ready-made polenta (about 16 ounces, cut into
    ½-inch-thick rounds)

Preheat grill to medium-high heat. Brush tops of eggplant slices with olive oil, drizzle garlic cloves with olive oil and sprinkle lightly with salt. Place garlic on a small sheet of foil. Place vegetables on the grill and roast until eggplant and garlic are golden brown and soft, about 15 minutes, turning eggplant slices to brown. If any pieces become too dark before all are done, remove them first. Cool slightly and then dice eggplant. While roasted garlic is still warm, place it into the bowl of a food processor fitted with a metal blade. Add capers, anchovies, thyme, rum and tomatoes and puree until it is still a little chunky. By hand, stir in eggplant and bell peppers. Stir in chopped parsley and a pinch of salt. Taste for seasoning. Reserve and keep warm. Brush polenta with olive oil and place on grill along with eggplant if space allows. Let brown and flip over so second side is brown. Brown all of the slices. Place on serving plate or platter and top with eggplant mixture. Sprinkle with more chopped parsley.

CALORIES	177
FAT	4 GRAMS
CALCIUM	2 MG
FIBER	3 GRAMS

SZECHWAN SPHERES

Inspired by Asian-style cuisine, these versatile patties are as flavorful as they are simple. The recipe can also be used for hors d'oeuvres by shaping the mixture into small spheres and baking for about 8 minutes. The spiciness of the dish can be adapted for low or high heat by adjusting the amount of cayenne pepper. For me, the spicier the better!   Serves 4

½ cup water chestnuts, finely chopped
⅓ cup scallions, finely chopped
½ cup celery, finely chopped
3 cloves garlic, finely chopped
1 cup cooked white rice
12 ounces ground chicken, turkey or pork
2 tablespoons grated fresh ginger
1 teaspoon sesame oil
½ teaspoon cayenne pepper (optional)
1 tablespoon orange marmalade
2 tablespoons soy sauce
3 tablespoons sesame seeds

Heat the oven to 425 degrees. Grease a sheet baking pan. In a large bowl, mix all of the ingredients together, except sesame seeds, and stir until well blended. Form into 4-inch-wide and 1-inch-high flat round patties. Sprinkle evenly with sesame seeds, pressing lightly to make them adhere. Place patties on the greased baking sheet and bake for 10 to 14 minutes, or until done in the center but not too dry. Place two patties on each plate and serve immediately.

CALORIES	229
FAT	7 GRAMS
CALCIUM	10 MG
FIBER	2.1 GRAMS

SPICY PUNJABI STEAK

A simple but pungent treatment for steak makes great use of time and creates an amazing flavor. This marinade can be made up in larger batches and kept refrigerated as an exotic barbecue sauce. Marinate the steak the night before cooking or in the morning before going to work. Serves 4

    3 cloves garlic, minced
    1 teaspoon curry powder
    1 tablespoon ginger, freshly grated
    3 tablespoons soy sauce
    3 tablespoons fresh lime juice
    1 tablespoon honey
    2 tablespoons cocktail sauce
    1 pound sirloin steak, cut 1 inch thick and trimmed of all fat

In a flat nonreactive bowl, mix all of the ingredients except steak. Add steak and let marinate for at least 8 hours. Heat a grill or broiler and cook steak to medium, turning halfway through cooking. Slice steak and divide evenly among four plates.

CALORIES	254
FAT	7 GRAMS
CALCIUM	3 MG
FIBER	0.4 GRAM

RED SNAPPER WITH BRANDY AND MIXED WILD MUSHROOMS

Mixed wild mushrooms and brandy make an elegant and simple complement for a delicate white fish such as red snapper, orange roughy or even farm-raised catfish. You can obtain the same earthy flavor and reduce costs if you substitute dried mushrooms—just soak for 30 minutes before using. Serves 4

    4 6-ounce red snapper fillets
    Salt and freshly ground pepper to taste
    ¼ cup all-purpose flour
    1 tablespoon olive oil
    1 medium onion, minced
    ⅓ cup flat-leaf parsley
    ½ cup fresh mixed wild mushrooms (such as shiitake, oyster,
        chanterelles or porcini) or dried mushrooms, rehydrated
        to yield ½ cup

¼ cup brandy
½ cup fish broth or clam juice

Season fish with salt and pepper, then dust with flour. In a large skillet over medium-high heat, add olive oil and heat until sizzling. Add onion and sauté for 1 minute. Add fish and cook for 2 minutes on each side or until lightly browned. Add 2 tablespoons of parsley, followed by mushrooms. Then add brandy and ¼ cup of fish broth. Flip snapper again and add remaining broth. Transfer fish and mushrooms to a platter or individual serving plates, pouring pan juices over them. Garnish with remaining parsley.

CALORIES	334
FAT	15 GRAMS
CALCIUM	6 MG
FIBER	0.8 GRAM

SALMON WITH PINEAPPLE WASABI

When an evening meal is in the works with no time to spare, throw together this fiery salmon recipe that is bold in flavor and low in fat. Wasabi powder (that hot green paste served with sushi) creates the flame, but prepared horseradish can also be used. Serve ramen or soba noodles made from buckwheat around the salmon.   Serves 4

4 4-ounce center-cut salmon fillets
1 6-ounce can crushed pineapple, drained
2 tablespoons honey
½ teaspoon Asian (toasted) sesame oil
1 tablespoon ginger, freshly grated
½ teaspoon Wasabi powder or 1 teaspoon horseradish
1 tablespoon soy sauce

Heat oven to 425 degrees. Line a sheet pan with foil. Place salmon fillets on the foil. In a small bowl, mix remaining ingredients together. Spoon mixture over the top of salmon fillets. Bake for 15 minutes.

CALORIES	263
FAT	13 GRAMS
CALCIUM	1 MG
FIBER	0.2 GRAM

CRISPY NOODLE CAKE WITH SHRIMP AND SUGAR SNAP PEAS

Transform plain old cooked spaghetti into a crispy noodle cake topped with a mild Asian shrimp and vegetable sauce. The trick for crisping the noodle cake is a good nonstick skillet, medium heat and patience. Don't peek too often—the bottom of the cake takes a while to thoroughly brown.   Serves 6

4 cups cooked spaghetti or capellini
1 tablespoon vegetable oil
2 teaspoons Asian (toasted) sesame oil
1 egg, lightly beaten
1 tablespoon ginger, freshly grated
2 cups chicken broth
2½ tablespoons cornstarch
3 tablespoons soy sauce
1 teaspoon sugar
1 teaspoon Asian (toasted) sesame oil
1 tablespoon vegetable oil
12 ounces medium shrimp (about 25), peeled, deveined,
     rinsed and patted dry
½ pound sugar snap peas, stems removed
3 tablespoons minced scallion
1½ tablespoons ginger root, peeled and minced

In a bowl, toss noodles with oils, egg and ginger. Heat a medium nonstick skillet on medium-high heat. Add noodle mixture, pressing gently to form a pancake in the skillet. Cook for 6 to 8 minutes without touching, or until the bottom of the cake is brown and crispy. Flip noodle cake and continue cooking until other side is crispy. Slide off onto a serving platter and hold at a warm temperature. Meanwhile, place chicken broth in a medium bowl and stir in cornstarch, soy sauce, sugar and sesame oil. In a wok or skillet, heat 1 tablespoon vegetable oil over high heat until it just begins to smoke. Add shrimp and stir-fry for 1 to 2 minutes, or until shrimp are just cooked through. Stir in broth mixture and simmer, stirring, for 1 minute. Add sugar snap peas, scallion and ginger and heat the mixture, stirring, until hot (about 1 minute). Pour the sauce over the noodle cake and serve by cutting into wedges.

CALORIES	334
FAT	9 GRAMS
CALCIUM	6 MG
FIBER	2.7 GRAMS

NORTH AFRICAN STEW

An adaptation from Bon Appétit *magazine, this recipe gives an exotic character to those vegetables that frequent our markets in the cold months but get little appreciation. The dish has been revised to work for our fast-paced schedule and is a meal in itself. It is greatly enhanced by a side dish of couscous garnished with toasted pepitas (pumpkin seeds) and scallions.* Serves 6

1 pound sweet potatoes, skin scrubbed
2 parsnips, peeled
8 ounces turnips or rutabagas, peeled
1 pound chicken thighs, boneless, skinless, and cut into
   1-inch cubes
1 cup onion, chopped
2 cloves garlic, minced
1 tablespoon fresh ginger, minced
1 teaspoon ground cumin
½ teaspoon cinnamon
½ cup chicken broth
1 16-ounce can diced tomatoes
Pepitas, toasted, for garnish
Scallions, shredded, for garnish

Place sweet potatoes, parsnips and turnips on a microwave-safe plate and microwave for 6 minutes to soften. Cut vegetables into ½-inch cubes. In a glass pie plate or bowl, place vegetables, chicken, onion, garlic, ginger, cumin, cinnamon, broth and tomatoes. Mix with a spoon. Cover with plastic wrap and microwave for 16 to 20 minutes, rotating twice during cooking. Vegetables should be soft and chicken pieces well done, but not dry. Stir and serve over a bed of couscous. Sprinkle the couscous with toasted pepitas and shreds of scallions. Serve immediately.

CALORIES	308
FAT	LESS THAN 1 GRAM
CALCIUM	26 MG
FIBER	6.5 GRAMS

HUEVOS RANCHEROS

Eggs for dinner? Why not—especially when they're part of a stacked Mexican classic that takes less than 20 minutes to build. Huevos (eggs) are one of those favorites that are complete meals in themselves. For any of the ingredients, the lower-fat variety is fine.

Serves 4

RANCHERO SAUCE

1 tablespoon olive oil
1 small onion, thinly sliced
1 small red or yellow bell pepper, thinly sliced
Dash hot sauce or 1 to 2 chipolte chiles, finely chopped
3 cloves garlic, minced
2 cups tomato sauce
1 teaspoon oregano
½ teaspoon cumin

1 tablespoon olive oil
8 eggs, lightly beaten
1 cup black beans, rinsed and drained
Salt and freshly ground pepper, to taste
4 6-inch flour tortillas, warmed
¾ cup shredded Monterey Jack pepper cheese
2 tablespoons fresh cilantro, chopped (optional)
Light sour cream for garnish

Put 1 tablespoon of olive oil in a medium skillet over medium-high heat. When hot, add onions and bell pepper and saute for 5 minutes. Add hot sauce, garlic, tomato sauce, oregano and cumin and heat until just bubbling. Lower heat to medium and simmer for 5 minutes. In a second medium skillet, heat remaining 1 tablespoon olive oil over medium-high heat. Add eggs and stir to mix until softly formed and creamy. Remove from heat, stir in black beans and salt and pepper to taste. Hold to keep warm. For each serving, place a warm flour tortilla on a serving plate. Top with a portion of scrambled eggs and a large spoonful or two of sauce. Sprinkle with shredded cheese and garnish with cilantro. Pass sour cream.

CALORIES	455 (without the sour cream)
FAT	18 GRAMS (without the sour cream)
CALCIUM	20 MG (without the sour cream)
FIBER	6.9 GRAMS (without the sour cream)

ARTICHOKE-STUFFED CHICKEN BREASTS

I was so inspired by the World Class Cuisine Cookbook *(Rutledge Hill Press, 1993) that I've adapted this recipe to help really whittle away those last 10!*   Serves 6

Salt and freshly ground pepper, to taste
6 4-ounce chicken breasts
1 clove garlic
1½ cups frozen or canned artichoke hearts, rinsed and
    drained
¼ cup egg substitute
2 tablespoons light sour cream
1 cup fresh bread crumbs
Dash nutmeg
⅓ cup fresh parsley, chopped; reserve 2 tablespoons
    for garnish
¼ cup chicken broth
Paprika

Heat the oven to 425 degrees. Grease a baking pan. Salt and pepper chicken breasts. Remove the fillet from each breast and reserve for the filling. With a very sharp, small knife, cut a pocket horizontally into each breast. Do not cut in half. Set aside while making the stuffing. In a food processor or Osterizer blender, place removed chicken breast fillets, garlic, artichoke hearts, egg substitute, sour cream, bread crumbs, nutmeg and about ¼ cup parsley. Process to mix, but do not puree. Place 2 to 3 tablespoons of stuffing in each breast pocket. Do not close the pocket—stuffing will puff up and out a bit. Place stuffed breasts on the baking sheet. Pour chicken broth over chicken. Sprinkle with paprika. Bake for 12 to 15 minutes. Place chicken breasts on a platter, spoon the pan juices over chicken and sprinkle with reserved parsley.

CALORIES	238
FAT	4 GRAMS
CALCIUM	7 MG
FIBER	2.4 GRAMS

TUSCAN TURKEY BREASTS WITH OLIVES

I love the style of Under the Tuscan Sun, *by Frances Mayes—it makes me ravenous! I was so inspired, I re-created her recipe, but adapted it for a crowd. Warn everyone if the olives have not been pitted!*   Serves 4

2 tablespoons olive oil
8 2-ounce turkey breast cutlets
1 medium onion, finely chopped
2 cloves garlic, minced
1 cup vermouth
Juice of 1 lemon
1 cup mixed green and black olives, pitted
Salt and freshly ground pepper, to taste
2 tablespoons fresh flat-leaf parsley, chopped

In a large skillet, heat 1 tablespoon of olive oil until hot over medium-high heat. Add turkey cutlets and sauté, quickly turning and cooking until almost done. Remove to a platter to keep warm. Add another tablespoon olive oil and then add onion and garlic and sauté for 2 minutes. Add vermouth, reduce the heat to low, cover and cook for 3 minutes. Return turkey to the pan and add the lemon juice and olives. Adjust salt and pepper seasoning and simmer for 5 minutes, or until turkey is done. Stir in a handful of parsley and serve.

CALORIES	288
FAT	13 GRAMS
CALCIUM	6 MG
FIBER	1.9 GRAMS

CAESAR PORK TENDERLOIN

We all love Caesar dressing! Now try my Caesar-infused pork dish, which lowers the calorie count and is so simple. Make a quick dressing with the traditional seasonings and wrap the coated tenderloin in Parmesan bread crumbs. Quick and tasty— my favorite type of "fast food."   Serves 4

Salt and freshly ground pepper to taste
1 16-ounce pork tenderloin
½ cup nonfat or low-fat mayonnaise
½ teaspoon anchovy paste
2 teaspoons fresh lemon juice

1 clove garlic, minced
1 cup crushed crouton crumbs
¼ cup freshly grated Parmesan cheese

Heat the oven to 425 degrees. Salt and pepper tenderloin. Combine mayonnaise, anchovy paste, lemon juice and garlic. On a plate, combine crouton crumbs and Parmesan. With a knife, spread mayonnaise mixture completely over tenderloin and then roll in crumbs to coat. Place on a flat baking sheet. Bake for 15 to 20 minutes or until tenderloin is medium-well (slightly pink in the center). Cut into ¼-inch-thick slices to serve.

CALORIES	272
FAT	12 GRAMS
CALCIUM	9 MG
FIBER	0.1 GRAM

Snacks

DENISE'S FAVORITE SWEET POTATO SNACK

Serves 4

2 medium-size sweet potatoes

Preheat oven to 350 degrees. Bake sweet potatoes until cooked (about an hour). If you're using a microwave, cook for about 15 minutes. Let potatoes cool, then cut in half and wrap each half in foil. Place in the refrigerator for 30 minutes or until cold. Serve potato halves in foil and eat with a spoon, like you're scooping your favorite ice cream out of a cone. Simple, nutritious and sweet!

CALORIES	58
FAT	0.05 GRAM
CALCIUM	16 MG
FIBER	1.7 GRAMS

DENISE'S GUILT-FREE SHAKES

A great calcium boost—even Jeff loves these low-calorie "milk" shakes!   Serves 4

1¼ cups nonfat milk
1 cup nonfat or low-fat vanilla yogurt
2 teaspoons vanilla

Place all ingredients in an Osterizer blender and process until smooth. Serve cold.

CALORIES	93
FAT	1 GRAM
CALCIUM	20 MG
FIBER	0 GRAMS

Need a little extra flavor? Try these variations:
Chocolate Shake: Add 2 tablespoons Ovaltine.
Strawberry Shake: Substitute strawberry yogurt for vanilla yogurt and add 2 cups sliced and hulled fresh or frozen strawberries.
Banana Shake: Substitute strawberry-banana yogurt for vanilla yogurt and add 2 cups sliced banana.

FLORIDA SPRITZER

A refreshing twist to a traditional summer cooler.   Serves 4

1½ cups Florida grapefruit juice
¼ cup sugar
2-inch cinnamon stick
Ice cubes
2 12-ounce cans ginger ale, chilled

For syrup: In a saucepan combine grapefruit juice, sugar and cinnamon. Bring to a boil; reduce heat. Simmer, uncovered, for 5 minutes. Discard cinnamon stick; cool syrup. Cover and chill syrup. To serve, fill four 8-ounce glasses with ice. Add about ⅓ cup grapefruit syrup to each glass. Fill glasses with ginger ale. Stir gently. If desired, garnish with Florida grapefruit curls, edible flowers and fresh mint sprigs.

DENISE'S HAPPY SNACKS

Snacking keeps your energy high, your metabolism revved and your stomach from growling. Here are some of my favorites!

Each snack serves 1

- 2 low-fat vanilla wafer sandwiches (4 cookies), each with ½ teaspoon low-fat cream cheese and 1 slice banana

- 2 tablespoons canned fat-free refried beans, microwaved on 1 6-inch tortilla

- 4 slices melba toast, each spread with 1 teaspoon nonfat cottage cheese with pineapple

- 2 celery stalks stuffed with low-fat cream cheese and chives

- 4 cinnamon graham cracker squares, each spread with ½ teaspoon jam

- 1 box Cracker Jack and ½ glass skim milk with 1 teaspoon chocolate Ovaltine

- 1 cup baby carrots dipped in nonfat cottage cheese mixed with salsa

Appendix A
The Best Bone-Boosting Snacks

Here are some super souces of calcium that you can include in your healthy home-cooked meals or nibble as snacks. Since most Americans don't get enough of this bone-building mineral, I recommend working these foods into your diet regularly. They're especially important for breast-feeding moms, who need extra calcium to support milk production.

Snack: **Low-fat yogurt**
Amount: 1 cup (8 ounces)
Calcium: 400 mg
Calories: 100–200

Snack: **Calcium-fortified orange juice**
Amount: 1 cup (8 ounces)
Calcium: 300 mg
Calories: 112

Snack: **Cheddar cheese**
Amount: 1 ounce (about
    1 domino-size piece)
Calcium: 204 mg
Calories: 170

Snack: **Frozen yogurt**
Amount: ½ cup
Calcium: 200 mg
Calories: 90–210

Snack: **Navy beans, cooked**
Amount: 1 cup
Calcium: 128 mg
Calories: 296

Snack: **Almonds**
Amount: 1 ounce (2 tablespoons)
Calcium: 90 mg
Calories: 170

Snack: **Skim milk**
Amount: 1 cup (8 ounces)
Calcium: 302 mg
Calories: 86

Snack: **Tofu set with calcium**
Amount: ½ cup
Calcium: 258 mg
Calories: 183

Snack: **Calcium-fortified cereal**
Amount: 1 cup
Calcium: 200 mg
Calories: 100–150

Snack: **Soybeans**
Amount: 1 cup cooked
Calcium: 175 mg
Calories: 298

Snack: **Broccoli**
Amount: 1 cup, cooked
Calcium: 72 mg
Calories: 44

Snack: **Frozen waffles**
Amount: 2
Calcium: 80 mg
Calories: 180–220

Appendix B
Fiber Food Swap

Ever since you saw your grandmother drinking prune juice, you've known that fiber is good for you. But you may not know exactly *how* good.

High-fiber foods such as prunes or bran cereal help keep you "regular," which is why many people eat them. But accumulating research shows that fiber does much, much more than aid digestion. High-fiber diets have been linked to a significantly lower risk of heart disease. Fiber provides a feeling of comfortable fullness, so you don't overeat. And it speeds the progress of food through your intestines before all of it can be absorbed and stored as fat. For each gram of fiber consumed, you can subtract about *nine calories* from your total calorie intake, researchers say.

The National Research Council estimates that the average American consumes about 12 grams of fiber per day—far less than the 25 to 40 grams recommended by many health-care practitioners. By following the meal plans in this book, you'll be getting a healthy 25 grams of fiber per day. After my four-week plan is over, you can use the following list to help you make healthy higher-in-fiber food choices:

Breakfast

INSTEAD OF:

1 cup of corn flakes: 1 gram fiber

White toast: 0–1 gram fiber

6 ounces of orange juice: 0 grams fiber

CHOOSE:

½ cup of Fiber One cereal: 13 grams fiber

Whole-wheat bread: 2–3 grams fiber

1 orange: 3 grams fiber

Lunch

INSTEAD OF:

A cheeseburger: 0 grams fiber

1 cup of chicken noodle soup: 2 grams fiber

A turkey sandwich on white bread: 1 gram fiber

CHOOSE:

Black bean burger: 4.8 grams fiber

1 cup of lentil soup: 5 grams fiber

⅓ cup hummus on a whole-wheat pita: 9 grams fiber

Snacks

INSTEAD OF:

Chips: 0 grams fiber

Cheese curls: 0 grams fiber

Gummi bears: 0 grams fiber

CHOOSE:

Baked tortilla chips with salsa: 2.2 grams fiber

Popcorn: 4.7 grams fiber

An oat-fruit granola bar: 1.7 grams fiber

Dinner

INSTEAD OF:

Marinara sauce: 3 grams fiber

⅔ cup of white rice: 0 grams fiber

Grilled chicken: 0 grams fiber

CHOOSE:

Chunky vegetable sauce: 6 grams fiber

⅔ cup of brown rice: 2.3 grams fiber

Veggie burger: 4 grams fiber

Appendix C
Healthy Food Swap

Breakfast

INSTEAD OF:	CHOOSE:
A large bagel	Half a bagel or 3.5-inch-diameter bagel
Regular latte	Skim-milk latte
NOTHING	Yogurt with fruit and a slice of whole-grain toast

Lunch

INSTEAD OF:	CHOOSE:
A whole sandwich	Half a sandwich and a cup of vegetable soup
Salad with fat-free dressing	Salad with 3 ounces of tuna and a mini-pita
Chicken salad croissant from the deli	Grilled chicken on a whole-grain bagel with tomato

Snacks

INSTEAD OF:	CHOOSE:
Twizzlers	Raisins
Ice-cream cone	Small soft-serve frozen yogurt on a cake cone
Rice cakes	A cup of mixed multigrain cereal and dried fruit

Dinner

INSTEAD OF:	CHOOSE:
Hand-size amount of meat	Palm-size amount of meat
Full plate of pasta	Half a plate of pasta and half of vegetables
Plain steamed veggies	Try grilled or roasted veggies for a taste change

About the Author

At 5 feet 4 inches and 112 pounds, Denise Austin has been dubbed "America's favorite fitness expert." From 1984 to 1988, Denise was the resident fitness expert on NBC's *Today* show. She also wrote a column for the *Washington Post* and received a prestigious award from the President's Council on Physical Fitness and Sports.

In 1987, Denise created her ESPN television show, *Getting Fit.* Today she is seen on Lifetime television's *Denise Austin's Daily Workout* and on her new show, *Denise Austin's Fit and Lite.* Her television show, which has aired for more than fifteen years, is rated number one and is seen in eighty-two countries. She is also the fitness expert of PBS's weekly television show *Health Week* and has her own Web site (deniseaustin.com).

Denise has created more than thirty best-selling exercise videos and has her own line of activewear and workout equipment. She was honored with the distinguished alumna award of 1997 by her alma mater and gave the commencement address to the graduates. She is an honorary board member of former Surgeon General C. Everett Koop, M.D.'s "Shape Up America" and has been appointed by two governors of Virginia as chairman of the governor's Commission on Physical Fitness and Sports.

Denise's sensible, realistic and enthusiastic approach to fitness (she works out only 30 minutes a day) and eating (she never skips a meal) has won fans throughout the United States, from whom she receives over 700 letters a week. But Denise believes her greatest achievement yet is being a mom to her two daughters, Kelly and Katie.

WHATEVER YOUR GOAL MAY BE, DENISE AUSTIN HELPS YOU GET THERE.

Don't miss these best-selling DVD & videos from America's favorite fitness expert, **Denise Austin!**

Available at your local video retailer

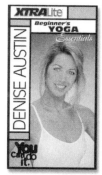

Denise Austin's Xtralite Beginner's Yoga Essentials
A selected variety of 4 basic Yoga routines that builds strength and stamina, promotes a healthy back and invigorates for a natural body tune-up. For focus and a renewed sense of well-being, it's Yoga Essentials.
Item # 893

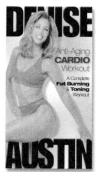

Denise Austin's Anti-Aging Cardio Dance Workout
A rejuvenating aerobic dance workout that will boost your metabolism and re-shape your entire body. One of the best videos for toning and firming muscles and shrinking that "middle-age spread."
Item # 962

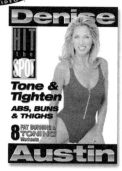

Denise Austin's Hit The Spot Tone & Tighten Abs, Buns, & Thighs
Tone, tighten and burn at the touch of a finger! Denise Austin's first workout on DVD featuring her most effective Hit The Spot routines, a relaxing mind/body cool down, plus a special "Ask Denise" chapter.
Item # 5534

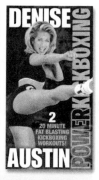

Denise Austin's Power Kickboxing
One of the hottest workouts from Denise! Combines a comfortably-paced, low-intensity workout while teaching the fundamentals of kick boxing during a non-stop, fat-burning aerobic routine. Kick, jab and punch away inches as you boost metabolism, increase energy and build strength.
Item # 832

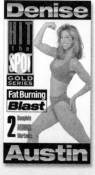

Denise Austin's Fat Burning Blast
One of Denise's best-selling titles ever! Two complete workouts featuring a low impact aerobic routine followed by an interval/circuit workout for toning and sculpting the muscles.
Item # 193

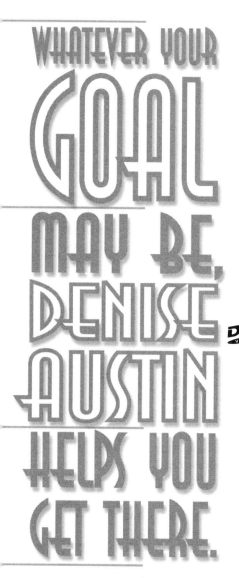